THE VITAMIN CURE

for Digestive Disease

DAMIEN DOWNING, MD
ANNE PEMBERTON, PGCE, RGN

ANDREW W. SAUL, PHD
SERIES EDITOR

T0273615

Basic Health
PUBLICATIONS, INC.

The information contained in this book is based upon the research and personal and professional experiences of the authors. It is not intended as a substitute for consulting with your physician or other healthcare provider. Any attempt to diagnose and treat an illness should be done under the direction of a healthcare professional.

The publisher does not advocate the use of any particular healthcare protocol but believes the information in this book should be available to the public. The publisher and authors are not responsible for any adverse effects or consequences resulting from the use of the suggestions, preparations, or procedures discussed in this book. Should the reader have any questions concerning the appropriateness of any procedures or preparation mentioned, the authors and the publisher strongly suggest consulting a professional healthcare advisor.

Basic Health Publications, Inc.
28812 Top of the World Drive
Laguna Beach, CA 92651
949-715-7327 • www.basichealthpub.com

Library of Congress Cataloging-in-Publication Data

Downing, Damien.
   The vitamin cure for digestive diseases / Damien Downing, MD,
Anne Pemberton, PGCE, RGN.
      pages cm
   Includes bibliographical references and index.
   ISBN 978-1-59120-367-4
   1. Digestive organs—Diseases—Alternative treatment. 2. Vitamin therapy.
I. Pemberton, Anne. Title.
   RC802.D79   2014
   616.3—dc23
                                                    2014029820

Editor: Karen Anspach
Typesetting/Book design: Gary A. Rosenberg
Cover design: Mike Stromberg

Printed in the United States of America

10   9   8   7   6   5   4   3   2   1

CONTENTS

Acknowledgments, v

Foreword, vi

CHAPTER 1. Are You Down in the Mouth? 1

CHAPTER 2. Reflux, aka GERD, 17

CHAPTER 3. Ulcers and *Helicobacter Pylori,* 37

CHAPTER 4. The Liver, 47

CHAPTER 5. The Biliary Tree, 57

CHAPTER 6. The Pancreas, 75

CHAPTER 7. Dysbiosis, 85

CHAPTER 8. Leaky Gut, 93

CHAPTER 9. The Large Intestine and Its Goings On or Out, 109

Action Plan, Section 1: Nutritional Approach, 121

Action Plan, Section 2: Supplements and Gallstone
                        Relief Program, 143

References, 167

Index, 173

About the Authors, 183

Acknowledgments

We would like to acknowledge Dr. Patricia Kane, as her work on essential fatty acids has greatly influenced the way we both practice. Dr. Kane had no hesitation, when asked, if we could share her recipes in this book. She has been happy to offer guidance and a different perspective on some of our most difficult cases. Thank you very much, Dr. Kane.

We would also like to acknowledge our artist, Janie Mason. Janie is a very special person who has recovered from Asperger's syndrome/ high functioning autism to the point that she runs her own tattoo parlor, paints, and sculpts. Her unique perspective on the art world is a breath of fresh air.

FOREWORD

The main thing you want from your digestive tract is that it does its job quietly, without talking back to you. You don't want to know that it's there.

That job is actually much bigger than you've ever imagined. Not only is the gastrointestinal system responsible for digesting and absorbing nutrients from food and for excreting waste, it is also the largest organ of your immune system. Over two-thirds of your body's lymphocytes (the captains of immune function) are found in the lining of the small intestine. From this base they travel throughout your body sending signals that influence immunity in all other organs.

Your gastrointestinal tract has its own nervous system, technically called the enteric nervous system (ENS) and affectionately dubbed "the second brain" by aficionados. Your ENS has as many nerve cells as your spinal cord and is in constant communication with your brain, impacting mood and cognitive function.

Your alimentary canal is also home to about a hundred trillion microbes, which include a thousand different species of bacteria and a few dozen types of yeasts. Collectively these are called the "gut microbiome." Understanding how these microbes influence human health and illness has been a major interest of mine for over three decades. In the last decade, microbiome research has blossomed into one of the most discussed topics in applied science. It's become clear that gut microbes help us to be human. The implications of that relationship will be at the cutting edge of clinical research for decades to come.

Finally, the gastrointestinal tract is an organ of detoxification. Most of this responsibility rests with the liver, but the intestinal lining is also rich in detoxifying enzymes. The liver and gut work together to remove noxious substances derived from food, your environment, gut microbes, and even the operation of your own metabolism and hormones.

These multiple functions of the digestive system interact with each other and with the food you eat to regulate your nutritional state, your metabolic state, your weight, your pattern of sleep, your energy, and your susceptibility to illness. *The Vitamin Cure for Digestive Disease* is a gold mine of practical information that allows you to help this system work for you, instead of against you.

Damien Downing has been a colleague and a leader in the field of nutritional medicine for over thirty years. The team of Downing and Pemberton has crafted a unique handbook that covers not only normal structure and function of the digestive system but helpful ways of treating a wide range of digestive disorders. Especially noteworthy components, which are often ignored in self-help books for digestive disorders:

- They start their discussion with the mouth, which is where digestion begins, and acknowledge the over arching impact of oral health on systemic health.

- They emphasize the importance of normal stomach acid and describe the many dangers of acid-suppressing drugs, the third largest-selling drug category in the world. For the past fifteen years, I've waged a campaign against acid suppressing drugs in the United States, where many powerful acid suppressors are available without a doctor's prescription. I created an e-book, *The Heartburn and Indigestion Solution,* to help people overcome their dependence on acid suppression.

- They give you strategies for dealing with the ulcer-causing bacterium, *H. pylori,* that go beyond standard drug therapy and are based on sound scientific evidence.

- They explain how to maintain a healthy liver and pancreas, the solid glandular organs that secrete into the digestive canal.

- They help you recognize the importance of small intestinal bacterial overgrowth, a disturbance in the ecology of the microbiome that allows normal bacteria to cause disease.

- In their timely discussion on the role of gluten and other fractions of wheat, they single out wheat germ agglutinin as a significant immune irritant. This key chemical is usually under the radar of popular books on nutrition.

- They explain the critical role of the intestinal lining as a barrier to toxins and allergens and give practical advice on reversing excessive intestinal permeability ("leaky gut").

- They call attention to the under-recognized role of nickel in food as an allergen and a disruptor of the normal intestinal barrier in sensitive individuals.

- They offer sound practical advice for controlling irritability and inflammation in the colon that goes beyond dietary fiber.

If you want to improve digestive health, *The Vitamin Cure for Digestive Disease* is an excellent place to start.

Leo Galland, MD, FACN, FACP
The Foundation for Integrated Medicine
Creator, www.pilladvised.com

CHAPTER 1

ARE YOU DOWN IN THE MOUTH?

We guess you are here to learn how to improve your digestive processes with good food and nutrition. To be honest, there is absolutely no point throwing in the vitamin pills if you don't adopt the healthy mouth approach and chew your food thoroughly. Food should be fluid when it moves from your mouth into your esophagus (the tube that runs from your mouth to your stomach through your throat), so if you are swallowing lumps when you eat then you certainly do need to read on. Your reason for swallowing your food in lumps might be laziness (I just want to get it down), timing (I only have fifteen minutes for lunch), or structural (I have ill-fitting dentures or missing teeth), or you may have an inflammatory condition of the mouth that is preventing you from chewing well and gaining all the possible goodness from the food you eat. We will be covering all of these in this chapter.

STRUCTURE AND FUNCTION OF THE MOUTH

The mouth or oral cavity is gaining popularity in terms of research. We have long been able to make a correlation between oral health and cardiovascular health, or, to be more precise, gum health and heart disease. However, we are beginning to see the mouth as the site of many chronic diseases. Some of these include dental caries (cavities), acquired immune deficiency syndrome (AIDS), periodontal disease (such as gingivitis), nutritional anemias, salivary gland disorders, osteoporosis, diabetes, and cancer. Congenital abnormalities are slightly different, however, they are generally related to poor maternal nutrient status, in particular folate deficiency.

The Teeth

To help you understand these relationships, we need to talk about teeth first. The teeth are a structure of enamel, dentin, and cementum wrapped around a nerve, which has huge blood supply. The teeth are retained in their bony sockets in the jaw by a fibrous structure called the periodontal membrane. Bacteria and inflammation can affect the integrity of this membrane, leading to tooth loss.[1]

Teeth are prone to nutrient deficiency even while the fetus is in utero (before birth, and well before teeth erupt through the gums), particularly of those nutrients that affect mineralization. Vitamin C has also been shown to affect tooth development and eruption. It is thought that this may be due to the action of vitamin C in collagen formation. If your vitamin C level is low, then bleeding and gum and bone disease may be the norm for you. Another interesting finding is that in areas of the world where goiter is endemic, children born to mothers with severe iodine deficiency are often born learning impaired, and their primary (baby or milk) teeth and secondary (permanent) teeth emerge very late. The teeth are likely to be maloccluded (crooked and misaligned) because the bone shape of the face and head are altered. This makes for a poor bite and the possibility of an inaccurate chewing mechanism.

Inside the Mouth

The mucosal surface of the mouth has a turnover rate of three to seven days. You could imagine the inside of the mouth and cheek as being analogous to a footpath. Wear and tear from many items of footwear (or the chewing of food particles) gradually thin down the top surface until it is so thin it literally becomes dust and sloughs off. While this is happening on the top surface the deep layers are replenishing and working their way to the top surface.

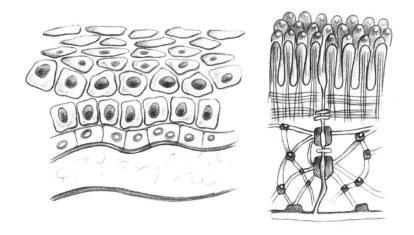

FIGURE 1.1. Diagram showing the layered structure of the cells inside the mouth (left). The image on the right is the inside of the cheek.

This means that a new surface is grown every seven days. Can you imagine the amount of energy required for the body to replicate cells this fast? Well, that energy has to come from somewhere. You need to eat nutrient-dense foods so that the specific nutrients required are pretty much on tap, so to speak. If there aren't enough available nutrients then DNA replication, protein synthesis, and cell maturation cannot occur. The barrier to toxic substances and oral microbes, and the antigens that would have been derived from these nutrients is lost, and infection can result. It doesn't take Einstein to work out that for this reason the mouth is the first region of the body to elicit signs of nutrient deficits and malnutrition.

To give you a few examples: A bright red, swollen, painful tongue may be an early sign of pernicious anemia, caused by a lack of vitamin B_{12}. Inflammation, tenderness, and/or burning of the tongue or inside of the mouth may be a sign of general vitamin B, protein, or iron deficiency. The inside of the mouth and tongue may become pale in an iron, folate, or vitamin B_{12} deficiency. A smooth, swollen tongue may indicate multiple nutritional deficiencies or malnutrition. Vitamin C deficiency manifests as red, swollen gums that bleed easily. Cracks in the corner of the mouth may also be due to vitamin B deficiencies, especially B_{12}. Please be aware, however, these descriptions are not diagnostic in any way. They are a signpost to finding out more. If you need more help, a good holistic dentist or doctor would be able to point you in the right direction.

We have focused on nutrient deficiency here, but we also need to consider overdosing with vitamins, which can also reduce the healing capacity of this delicate mucous membrane. You could also get rebound withdrawal after megadosing. Personally, we wouldn't recommend megadosing without professional help. Vitamins can become as toxic as drugs to the body if taken to excess.

The Function of the Mouth

Ok, so back to the function of this organ. The mouth is incredibly important for beginning the whole digestive process. What is sad is that we generally have this *laissez faire* attitude toward it. We throw all manner of things in it and expect it to keep on chewing. Well, that's if we know how to chew, and we do this act efficiently and effectively.

Before we get onto the chewing bit we will walk you through the structure and function of the mouth. This little guy is the first part of that long digestive tube we call the gastrointestinal (GI) tract. Digestion begins even before you take a bite. Think about your favorite meal: long before you get a taste, you can smell it being cooked, and your mouth starts watering. This moisture is saliva, and it contains amylase, an enzyme that helps to digest the starch in foods.

Have you ever chewed a piece of whole-grain bread for ages? If you haven't you should try it. The longer you chew starches the sweeter they get, and it's the amylase that does this for you. (Makes me wonder why we ever started adding sugar and sweeteners to foods for this very reason.) Starches are foods such as potato, bread, and pasta. In the laboratory these are known as polysaccharides or multichain sugars linked together. Salivary amylase starts to break up these links, turning the food into simple sugars ready for digestion, and that's why the food tastes sweeter the longer you chew. This is really important because simple sugars can be readily absorbed into the bloodstream once they get farther down the GI tract. The chewing and grinding action of teeth also helps to break down the fibers in the food, increasing the surface area for the enzymes to do their bit. This process is also really important for protein, as this food is fibrous and really hard to break down.

You have three pairs of salivary glands. Two pairs can be found in the floor of your mouth, more specifically, under the tongue and under the jawline; and another pair is situated one inside each cheek in front of each ear. This third pair can become swollen and inflamed. When they do we look a bit like a chipmunk, and we call this mumps. You may remember this from childhood, and if you are my age your mum would have sent you to the mumps party to "build up your immune system." Great fun that was, wasn't it—especially the after-effects ten days later.

You can think of the lining of the mouth as that footpath we mentioned above. It has many layers of flat cells, regenerating from the bottom layer. The layers eventually work their way to the top, where they die and slough off. This is good news because it means we can take swabs inside the mouth to put in a growing medium that will help us identify bacteria that may be causing a problem, or we can look at them under a microscope to see if the cells are behaving as they should.

The teeth and gums and upper and lower jaws (mandible and maxilla) provide the structure of the mouth, while a multitude of muscles allow all that chewing to happen. Saliva is continually produced to keep the pavement of the mouth lubricated. The roof of the mouth, called the palate, separates the mouth from the nasal cavity. It is hard at the front and soft at the back to allow swallowing. The palate is really important because it has a rich blood supply and a good nerve supply. The accessory nerve, responsible for supplying nerve input actually courses with the Vagus nerve. You will hear much more about this important nerve later when we talk about gastroesophageal reflux disease (GERD).

The tongue is one huge muscle attached to the structural bones of the mouth on all sides. This muscle is covered by mucous membrane to keep it nice and wet. It is important for taste, chewing, swallowing, and speech. The muscles of the mouth get the most exercise of any muscle in the body (and that figures).

So what about the teeth? Well, the optimum situation is a perfect set of well-aligned teeth in healthy gums. Interestingly, in the United States 57 percent of people over sixty-five wear dentures. Unless these are a perfect fit that's a huge percentage of the population who can no longer eat *al dente* and certainly will have difficulties with the old nutritional powerhouse standby of nuts and seeds. This most certainly limits the amount of nutrients that can be gained from the food they eat. We know loads of lovely old folk who want to help themselves towards better health by choosing healthier foods and cooking options. Asking them to steam their veggies just means they leave the steamer on for an hour. No point in that if good nutrition is the goal, but at least they enjoy casseroles and stews, with which we lose fewer nutrients. Don't despair if you are one of the 57 percent. We do have a solution for you in the digestion plan at the end of the book.

Another interesting fact is that in Chinese medicine each tooth has a corresponding organ in the body, attached by an energy system called a meridian. The Chinese speak a lot of sense and their approaches are rooted in centuries of medical research. They claim that if a tooth is affected by infection such as an abscess then its corresponding organ will also be affected. (We haven't got the space to go into this in detail, but we would recommend that you perform a Google search for "teeth meridians.") The natural dentists really have this covered so you can easily print off a chart for your kitchen wall. Teeth are classified as incisors (four upper and four lower) or front teeth, four canines (eyeteeth), eight premolars, and twelve molars. The teeth are shaped for purpose, so this should give clues as to their function. The incisors break off or cut food, the canines help with the cutting, and the premolars and molars help with the crushing and grinding to make solid food into a liquid bolus ready for swallowing. Interestingly, the upper molars are very close to the maxillary sinus that spans between the nose and eye, so any infection in these teeth can cause sinusitis, and sinusitis can cause toothache. You will know if you have ever had this. Also, any infection or damage around the nerve of the tooth will undoubtedly result in a searing pain that travels up the route of the nerve, usually up the side of the head and hairline. We call this neuralgia, and the herpes virus is a common cause of this.[2] Herpes is one of those dreaded viruses that lays dormant until we have overworked, overstressed, or been ill without recovery time. If you suffer with this, dear friend, you will be well aware of the tell-tale tingle. We will come back to herpes later, but for now we will look at some of the other conditions that might prevent you from chewing well.

Aphthous Stomatitis

We know these as mouth ulcers—those ugly, shallow, and extremely painful sores we generally stick a bit of soothing gel on and ignore as much as we can. They are also called canker sores. The dictionary definitions for "canker" are "an open lesion caused by fungus or protozoan (single-celled organism)" and "a malign and corrupting influence that's difficult to eradicate." They are usually about 10 millimeters (mm) (.39 inches [in]) across and generally resolve in seven to twenty-one days. However, they are often not a once-in-a-lifetime event for many of us. They are not infectious to others, so kissing doesn't have to stop, although that too could be painful. They generally have a grayish center membrane and an intense red border. They affect around 20 percent of the population and can keep reoccurring, so we need to find the underlying cause. So what are the underlying causes?

• Anything that may cause friction could be at fault. So, being too heavy-handed with the toothbrush, wearing badly-fitting dentures, injury from slipping with that pencil you are chewing, recent dental work, or eating foods that are too hot or too spicy. It doesn't take much to damage the sensitive lining of the mouth and remove too many of those layers.

• Emotional stress or anxiety especially if it is chronic, as this depletes the immune system. A small-scale study was performed on dental students who had a single aphthous ulcer on the roof of their mouth. The ulcer took 40 percent longer to heal when the students were under the stress of exams. Interleukin 1, which is a protein that signals other immune cells, was 60 percent lower during the same period.[3]

- Changes in hormone levels. Some women find they are plagued with canker sores just before their period while others develop them postmenopause.

- Nutrient deficiency. The cells in the lining of the entire GI tract have such a rapid turnover (four days) that often the shedding of cells becomes disordered. This may be the first signal of nutrient deficiency. The key nutrients here are thiamine, iron, folate, vitamin B_{12}, and zinc. Several studies have identified a causal association. Others have also associated pyridoxine and riboflavin. What is clinically interesting is that intramuscular B_{12} can eradicate both cold sores and canker sores in a few hours.

Nutrient deficiency can often be seen first in the mouth due to its high turnover of cells. Low levels of transketolase (a thiamine-dependent enzyme) have been found in those with recurrent aphthous stomatitis. Low levels of iron, folate, or vitamin B_{12}, or any combination of these were found in 14.2 percent of sufferers. This also links to poor methylation, so it could be one link between oral health and cardiovascular disease. Also, 28.2 percent were found to be deficient in vitamins B_1, B_2, or B_6 and were found to completely reverse their aphthous stomatitis once these levels were corrected. Zinc, given at 50 milligrams (mg) daily for one month, has been shown to reverse aphthous stomatitis and keep it in remission for a further three months.

- We will not be going into great detail here on the subject of allergies except to say that patients with celiac disease (discussed later) have high frequency of recurrent canker sores. (*The Vitamin Cure for Allergies,* another book in this series, covers this.) Studies designed to compare microscopic evaluation of lesions and white blood cell elevations have demonstrated a causal link. The two major culprits are gluten and casein.

- Environmental allergens: Preservatives such as benzoic acid, methylparaben, dichromate, and sorbic acid have been known to commonly induce canker sores.

- Too many refined foods in the diet.

Treatment for aphthous stomatitis includes:

- An elimination diet—to test for gluten and casein allergens.

- An alpha 1 gliadin antibody assay—to diagnose gluten sensitivity.

- Quercetin supplementation—inhibits mast cell degranulation, basophil histamine release, and the formation of other mediators of inflammation.

- DGL (deglycyrrhized licorice root) supplementation—DGL provides nutritional support for the GI tract, stimulates growth of mucus-secreting cells, and supports epithelial tissue and healthy cell function.

- Vitamin C supplementation—one of vitamin C's main functions is the manufacture of collagen, and, as collagen binds all cells to hold our bodies together, it is vital for wound repair and healthy gums.

- High-potency multivitamin supplementation—a multivitamin provides a baseline of overall nutritional support when it is clear that enough nutrients are not being gained from the diet.

Oral Thrush

This is a nasty infection caused by the *Candida albicans* fungus. You are more likely to experience this after repeated antibiotic use or if your immune system is struggling with other matters. For some it manifests as a result of prolonged stress or any another factor that impedes normal digestion. (You will learn more about this later, as this is what the book is all about.)

Thrush is the white-coated tongue you can see in those who are frail and ill. We really don't want to put you off your lunch, but it resembles cottage cheese. It can grow anywhere inside the mouth, but often you see it on the tongue, at the back of the mouth, and around the tonsils. There is lots of hype about a condition called candidiasis. We will cover this in more detail later, but for now just know that this little fungus likes the digestive tract and its warm, wet mucous membranes. If you have it then you know that it generally takes away the desire to eat rather than causing pain and suffering. That said, it can be very painful in some people. When it is sore it can seriously affect swallowing and chewing, limiting food choice and nutrition at a time when nutrition is needed the most.

In those with Crohn's or non-celiac gluten sensitivity, it is often very difficult to maintain adequate nutrition, and oral lesions can result. Other risk factors include the use of steroid inhalers, smoking, medications that reduce the saliva in the mouth, birth control pills, diabetes, poorly fitting dentures, iron or vitamin B deficiency, chemotherapy, radiotherapy, and excessive use of antibacterial mouthwashes, especially those that are alcohol based. Interestingly low levels of iron, folate, and/or vitamin B_{12} have been found in patients with oral thrush. You can buy antifungals over the counter, but the little blighter will keep bouncing back if you don't address the underlying causes.

Herpes Simplex

You will know this better as cold sores. It's a recurrent viral infection that attacks the skin or mucous membranes. There are a number of types, but we are really only concerned with two of them right now: herpes gingivostomatitis, which occurs inside the mouth; and herpes labialis, which occurs on the lip borders. Herpes simplex can start with one blister or a cluster of blisters that burst and spread. Those who suffer with herpes infections know only too well the pain of an outbreak. There are more than seventy members of the herpes family. Herpes simplex (HSV), varicella-zoster (VZV), Epstein-Barr (EPV), and *Cytomegalovirus* (CMV) are the four important ones in human disease. It is very difficult to treat viral infections as they lay dormant in human nerve cells until we overwork ourselves or succumb to the ravages of stress. Once the immune system is suppressed the telltale tingle appears, then the blister. If you are quick at catching the tingle you may be lucky and prevent the infection before it

ARE YOU DOWN IN THE MOUTH?

spoils your looks. It really isn't the right thing to tackle this with antiviral medication, although it may help in the short-term. The striking thing about herpes simplex is that it runs down the nerves, so whichever nerve is affected determines where the pain will be.

Supporting the immune system and reducing stress seems to be the magic potion for herpes. It's really important to support the thymus gland, and the key nutrients to do this are zinc, vitamin B_6, and vitamin C. When zinc is low the T helper cells, which are important for immune function, are reduced or fail to mature; thymic hormone levels diminish; and many of the actions of our white cells diminish with them.[4] Thymus extracts have also been highlighted as a potential treatment. Studies have shown that whether the ratio of T helper cells to T suppressor cells is high or low, thymus extracts may be of benefit,[5] as they appear to increase the immune system's response to herpes. Oral supplementation with zinc (50 mg per day) has been shown to reduce the frequency, duration, and severity of herpes outbreaks in clinical studies. The topical application of zinc sulphate has also shown promise.

Both oral and topical vitamin C can increase the rate of healing in herpes ulcers. In one randomized double blind study Asconal (a pharmaceutical grade ascorbic acid preparation) was applied with a soaked cotton-wool pad three times daily for two minutes. Researchers were much less able to culture herpes in cultures from the treatment group compared to the placebo group. In another study twenty subjects given 1,000 mg vitamin C with bioflavonoids outperformed subjects taking a placebo by 5.6 days.

Lysine and arginine are two amino acids that oppose each other in the body. Lysine has been shown to have antiviral activity due to blocking arginine. Foods high in arginine include chocolate, nuts, seeds, and almonds. Foods rich in lysine include vegetables, fish, legumes, and poultry. Long-term studies have shown mixed results, but that doesn't mean it won't work for you or that it isn't worth a try.

Topical applications that may confer benefit include lemon balm (*Melissa officinalis*), which should be applied to the lips two to four times per day. It can be applied fairly thickly. Another popular topical treatment is licorice (the root of *Glycyrrhiza glabra*). This is known to inhibit a number of viruses of which HSV is only one.

In addition to providing you with fresh breath, some studies have demonstrated that peppermint oil extract is superior to chlorhexidine mouthwash in inhibiting the biofilms associated with dental caries. In vitro peppermint has significant antimicrobial and antiviral qualities.[6]

Leukoplakia

Leukoplakia is a white lesionlike formation on the inside of the mouth. It grows like scar tissue, thick and hardened. It may not give you any symptoms until it cracks, but it is the precursor to cancer so it should be taken seriously. It has a tendency to occur in the fifty-to-seventy-year age group. Don't confuse this with lichen planus (described below), which can occur on both the mucosal surface and on the skin. The mouth is the most common place to find cancer, so now is the time to actively work to reduce this if you can. The most important thing to do is to stop smoking. The second thing to do is to improve your antioxidant status.

Both vitamin A and beta-carotene have been found clinically to be effective in controlling leukoplakia. The evidence of the protective effect of these nutrients against oral cancers is overwhelming.[7] There are other antioxidants that have also been studied. Some studies have shown that vitamin E can produce a 65 percent positive response rate. The important thing with vitamin E supplementation is to ensure you have a natural form of the vitamin, such as mixed tocopherols and tocotrienols.

Lichen Planus

As mentioned above, this condition frequently can be confused with leukoplakia in some people. The difference between the two is that lichen planus has a lacey effect and resembles lichen. It can grow anywhere on the body and can be confused with psoriasis. It is said to affect 27 people in 100,000, principally in the over-forty-five age group.[8] There are some schools of thought that believe lichen planus is triggered by shock, a virus, or biliary cirrhosis. (We discuss biliary tree difficulties later.) The good thing with lichen planus is that only

2 percent of cases develop oral cancer, so the risk is no greater than it is in the general population. It can resolve by itself, so often people delay that visit to their doctor.

Periodontal Disease

Do you have bleeding gums or gums that seem to be lifting away from the tooth? Does your bathroom sink resemble the Texas chain saw massacre when you brush your teeth? Is brushing your teeth uncomfortable due to sensitivity? If you are answering yes to any or all of these questions then you should be reading this part. Periodontal disease generally occurs as a result of infection, so it may be localized to the mouth. In this case it may be gingivitis (an infection of the gum line) or periodontitis (where the bone and ligaments attaching the tooth are destroyed, leading to the loss of perfect teeth).

We have put these guys together in one section, but they are indeed separate conditions. Both are caused by plaque formation, which allows bacteria to grow around the gum line, but the bacteria are different in each case. Gingivitis is relatively easy to treat, as it is more localized and superficial. Periodontitis is a slow and insidious disease. It can manifest as a result of underlying health problems. Inflammatory bowel disease such as Crohn's or celiac disease may cause periodontal disease. We will discuss these later, but they both create lots of inflammation in the body. Leaking amalgam fillings are another main cause, so you might want to find a mercury-free dentist to get those filings checked.

Our immune system is so busy on high alert when these types of conditions are present that it starts to get confused and attacks itself. The bacteria are then free to have a party on us! There isn't a lot of hard evidence pointing to autoimmune effects on oral health, and there are lots of promises for a "cure," so please be aware. Periodontal disease is so complex in some people that it may require professional help to get it stabilized. However, that doesn't mean we can't offer you what the latest research tells us can help.

Nutrient deficiency and malnutrition can allow inflammation to become exaggerated and cause wound healing to be very slow. This is mainly due to alterations in the antibacterial content of our saliva.

If you have type 1 or type 2 diabetes or osteoporosis, you are more likely to suffer with some degree of periodontitis. This is also true of conditions such as metabolic syndrome, cardiovascular disease (atherosclerosis, hypertension, or arrhythmias). These are all conditions caused by chronic inflammation. Even pregnancy or menopause can upset hormone ratios that may have an impact on periodontitis. By the time we add genetic predisposition to the list it looks like we are all prone!

Don't worry; once we tell you this bit we'll get your spirits back up again. All is not lost—but first we want to tell you a bit about diabetes and oral health. It's important to discuss this because a lot of you readers will be diabetic, and diabetes can have a profound effect on the mouth. If diabetes is not well controlled all of that glucose circulating in the bloodstream thickens up the blood, preventing nutrient absorption into the tissues. This excess glucose has to go somewhere, so it is absorbed into the body's tissues. In the case of the mouth, saliva can become sweet and sticky. Dysgeusia (taste distortion) may occur from an overgrowth of thrush (which feeds on glucose) or a zinc deficiency. Interestingly zinc plays a big part in the ability to taste and in quelling inflammation.

Here's a bit of an insight into osteoporosis (sorry if this doesn't apply, but we just want to link all of these potential underlying conditions together with periodontal disease. Those who have these conditions will then know that what they should do nutritionally for their main condition that should have some effect on their oral health). To be fair, the osteoporosis link is a strange one. There has been speculation in the medical literature for a long time that calcium deficiency and osteoporosis are underlying triggers for periodontitis. Some researchers say that periodontitis may be the first sign of systemic metabolic bone disorders such as this.[9] Given that currently 50 percent of women and 12.5 percent of men over sixty-five have osteoporosis, should we be paying more attention to this potential link and the underlying nutritional deficits? Anyway, the thing that is happening is this: When there is a negative calcium balance in the body, calcium is more easily mobilized from the skeleton, where there is trabecular bone. This is a softer, spongier bone found at the end of long bones. It is typically found in the hip joint and vertebrae, which of course take all the stress and bone loss. The alveolar process, or jawbone, is very similar. Studies have shown that women with severe postmenopausal osteoporosis are three times likely to have lost all their teeth.[10] Dietrich[11] also found that higher levels of vitamin D_3 were associated with a decrease in loss of tooth attachment in the over-fifty age group. So why are we telling you all this? Well, although it isn't absolutely crucial to have a full set of perfect teeth to maintain nutritional health, the loss of teeth or periodontium can have a profound effect on your food choices. The soreness, pain, tooth sensitivity, and tooth mobility can lead to a preference for foods of low nutritional value and a dependency on foods that require no chewing. Dentures can also pose difficulties. Hard foods such as nuts and seeds leach under the dentures to tear at the gums underneath. Does this mean you have to give up these little powerhouses of nutrients if you have these issues? Absolutely not! We will tell you how to bypass this hurdle at the end of the book.

CHAPTER 2

REFLUX, AKA GERD

So you have just been given a diagnosis of gastroesophageal reflux disease (GERD) from your gastroenterologist, or your general practitioner has mentioned GERD: what does it mean, exactly? You are going to need to know this in order to adequately manage your new friend although my guess is your GERD is not being so much of a friend at the moment. Don't be deterred by his unfriendliness. Read on for some insight into the possible causes for GERD's visit and a step-by-step guide to managing these underlying causes and the resulting symptoms. A good point to make here is that you are not alone. It is often said that up to 30 percent of the westernized population visit their doctor with symptoms related to GERD. Many more never visit their doctor but turn to complimentary practitioners because they recognize the cause and effect relationship that is occurring but cannot work it out on their own, or because they don't feel traditional Western medical practitioners have thoughtfully listened to them.

We are not here to choose one method of practice over the other or to paint a good-guy-bad-guy picture. We're here to give you sound advice so that you can hopefully make an informed choice that is manageable, and ultimately the correct choice for you. What we will tell you is that GERD and its treatments have been the target of aggressive marketing to both professionals and consumers. Proton pump inhibitors, the class of medications prescribed for GERD, are in fact the third best-selling drug worldwide. Sadly, they are merely a sticking plaster to cover the problem, instead of a true resolution of the cause. They can reduce the symptoms of GERD significantly, but this comes at a price. These drugs were meant for short-term use, but the rebound effects that occur when they are stopped generally leads to a dependency. With this comes the risk of stomach acid suppression and its resulting consequences, including osteoporosis, depression, vitamin B_{12} and mineral deficiencies, small intestinal bacterial overgrowth, irritable bowel syndrome, and *Clostridium difficile* infectious diarrhea. The latter can be life-threatening to the elderly. However we do have a catch-22 here in that untreated GERD can increase the risk for erosive esophagitis, Barrett's esophagus, and esophageal cancers. What clearly is needed is a new approach here, and the two questions we need to ask are:

1. "How and why has normal function been disturbed?"

2. "How can we assist the body to return to normal function?"

As you have probably guessed by now, there are ways to achieve this that will bring significant improvement and relief of symptoms. How cool would it be to take therapeutic foods and nutrients to do this? If you are game to try, then please read on.

STRUCTURE AND FUNCTION OF THE ESOPHAGUS

The esophagus, or gullet, is a muscular tube about nine inches long that begins in the throat and ends at the cardiac sphincter at the top end of the stomach. The cardiac sphincter, which some call the lower esophageal sphincter or the gastroesophageal sphincter, is a circular muscle around the bottom of the esophagus that opens for food to enter the stomach and closes to stop food from backflowing. You will see later that this particular sphincter is really important when it comes to GERD. The esophagus lies directly behind the main breathing tube, or bronchus, and in front of the spine. It is made up of three layers: the muscular layer, the areolar layer, and the mucous layer.

The muscular layer has fibers running down and around the esophagus in two separate layers. The outer layer is the longitudinal fiber that runs down the length of the esophagus. Beneath this layer are circular muscle fibers that run horizontally at the upper and lower ends of the esophagus and diagonally in the middle. This double layer of specific muscle arrangements allows the muscles to contract in sequence, creating waves (peristalsis). This moves the food bolus (from the Latin for "ball") along in the same way a worm moves along through the soil.

The areolar layer is a layer of connective tissue that literally provides the glue between the outer muscle layers and the inner mucous layer or membrane. This mucous layer is also very important because it houses many glands, particularly at the base of the esophagus around the all-important cardiac sphincter. These glands secrete mucus onto the surface of the membrane. This mucus protects the delicate mucous membrane from the acid of the stomach. How fantastic is it that the body protects itself in this way?

SO, WHAT IS GERD?

Well, GERD is a relatively new concept in terms of disease process, only really recognized in the last few years. Put very simply, GERD is the myriad chronic symptoms that originate from damage to the mucosal layer of the esophagus. As mentioned above, the mucosal layer is there to protect the structure of the esophagus from acid erosion. Damage occurs when the acid contents of the stomach are allowed to excessively or continuously backflow up the esophagus. In addition to stomach acids the stomach contents may also include bile acids, protein splitting enzymes (proteases), and pepsin. All of these substances can cause irritation and inflammation of the delicate esophageal lining. The end result of this backflow is:

- Heartburn—a burning sensation in your chest that sometimes spreads to the throat and sometimes is accompanied by a sour taste in your mouth.

- Chest pain—you need to seek medical help if you suffer chest pain with associated symptoms such as pain radiating to the left arm or jaw and shortness of breath.

- Difficulty swallowing (dysphagia)—this occurs more in age-related GERD and can give rise to aspiration pneumonia, a life-threatening situation in the elderly.

- Hoarseness or sore throat—in severe cases this may even be loss of the voice.

- Regurgitation of food or sour liquid (acid reflux)—likely to occur when bending forward or lying down after eating or when overeating. It also occurs more if you are heavier than normal.

- Sensation of a lump in your throat—this can be the result of swelling of the mucous membranes due to acid erosion or to build up of mucous as the body attempts to protect the throat.

Some of you may have one or more of these symptoms without really associating them with GERD.

Jo came to me (AP) with a ten-month history of severe hoarseness and loss of voice. As a telephone sales employee Jo was asked to leave her post on health grounds, being unable to speak and be understood on the telephone. Jo found it difficult to accept reflux as a cause without experiencing the symptom. Why was I so convinced? Jo was overweight for her height, skipping meals during the day then eating a huge meal at night and sometimes a heavy supper before retiring. She was also one of those people who curled up in a chair rather than sitting erect. Jo wasn't aware of the reflux because it was mostly occurring at night. The weight of Jo's excess belly fat was pushing up into her stomach, laden with food, weakening her lower esophageal sphincter. Jo slept so soundly she wasn't even aware. Losing some weight, eating little and often and significantly reducing convenience foods made a huge impact for Jo. This was an easy case, and I grant not every case will be this simple. So read on for more advice.

So we hope Jo's case has given you a good idea of the simple cases in life. That said we are all different beings and one size never fits all. Looking at Jo's case specifically, we can be misled into believing her overeating at night might overstimulate her gastric secretion of acid, leading to the reflux that cost her job. This would be a misconception. Clinical testing of stomach acidity (pH) has demonstrated that most people who suffer with reflux are found to have low levels of stomach acid or inappropriate timing of stomach acid secretion when there is no food in the stomach. Low stomach acid, or hypochlorhydria, creates an ideal environment for an opportunistic little bug called *Helicobacter pylori* to set up residence and cause havoc. Now I'm not going to go into much detail about this little guy here because he has a strong presence in another chapter of the book. What we will say here, though, is that if you have an ongoing problem with reflux then you need to rule out this bug as a cause. If he is living with you, then you are in luck right now if you go to the chapter on ulcers.

Let me explain what happens with hypochlorhydria. First of all, the foods you eat in any given meal or snack may make up any combination of carbohydrates, proteins, fats, or oils. Generally speaking, carbohydrates are easier to digest, proteins take longer, and fats even longer still. As we explained in the oral health chapter, chewing breaks up the fibers in the food, increasing the surface area so that appropriate digestive secretions can do the digestion and absorption processes for us. In the case of stomach acid, its primary role is to denature protein, breaking it down into amino acids for the body to use in building and repair work. If there isn't enough stomach acid to do this effectively then protein becomes difficult to digest. It may be obvious that food stays in the stomach too long, in other words, more than three hours. However, the other thing that happens is that the carbohydrates will become stagnant as they will stay in the stomach until the protein is digested and the food mass can move on. The low acid level then lets any opportunistic bacteria in the stomach have a party, fermenting the carbohydrates until a volcano erupts with a surge of stomach contents up into the esophagus. This is reflux. (Those of you used to brewing your own beer and/or wine will be familiar with this scenario.) That surge of stomach contents, despite its having a lower than normal level of stomach acid, can burn and irritate the delicate mucosa in the esophagus, and the symptoms are born.

So what other factors might also cause reflux, or the volcano eruption?

- Obesity—abdominal fat compresses the stomach contents, increasing intra-abdominal pressure.

- Pregnancy—over 50 percent of pregnant women are said to suffer reflux.

- Cigarette smoking—cigarettes are stimulants, which put the body into a stress response. This naturally reduces digestive secretions. In acute, temporary stress an adrenaline rush can save your life. However, constant, chronic stress shuts down digestion and this can require permanent support.

- Chocolate—high-fat, high-sugar foods such as chocolate are tough on the stomach and digestion. The fat takes hours to digest, leaving the sugars to ferment—and *voilà!* Another volcano.

- Too many fried foods—fats need proteins to allow them to be carried through the digestive processes. Too many fats with too little proteins leave a stomach full of fat, lying heavy.

- Carbonated drinks—already highly fermented, and absolute dynamite to an already fermenting gut.

- Alcohol—highly fermentable, and the relaxing effects come immediately, which is great for lower esophageal sphincter relaxation but bad for reflux.

- Coffee—a known gastric irritant and stimulant, so this works in the same way as cigarette smoking.

- Food intolerances—there are a number of known foods that are reputed to be causative factors for GERD. The commonly known ones include wheat and/or gluten, dairy, tomatoes, citrus, highly spiced foods, garlic, onions, and those foods already mentioned above.

- SIBO (small intestinal bacterial overgrowth)—potentially pathogenic bacteria upset the sensitive ecosystem of the small intestine, resulting in flatulence and bloating, and disruption of the normal transit time for digestion.

Long-Term Effects of GERD

We guess the burning question (pun intended) is, "why even bother about treating GERD when your doctor can give you a proton-pump inhibitor (PPI) pill and you can throw in some extra over-the-counter heartburn meds as needed?" A simple solution to a simple problem—or is it? In my opinion there are some really important reasons to take stock and work with this. Here are three specific long-term effects from having GERD:

1. Persistent or constant eruption of stomach contents or back pressure onto the lower esophageal sphincter can be the root cause of hiatal hernia. (We will discuss this in more depth a little later on.)

2. Persistent low levels of stomach acid can give rise to nutritional deficiencies and age-related pathologies or illnesses associated with these deficiencies.

3. Persistent GERD may cause such damage that it will require surgery.

4. There is a strong correlation between GERD and esophageal cancers.

We will discuss each of these in turn, so we will start with hiatal hernia.

Hiatus (Hiatal) Hernia

Remember our discussion about the gastroesophageal sphincter earlier in this chapter? Well, now we are going to talk about its neighbor, another muscle directly above it, that we call the diaphragm. The diaphragm is a huge fibrous muscle that lies in a horizontal plane, separating the thoracic or chest cavity (where your lungs are) from the abdominal cavity (or tummy). It prevents the organs of the abdomen, in particular the stomach, from rising up into the chest. It is also one of the important muscles in helping to maintain breathing. The esophagus travels through a small opening in the diaphragm (the hiatus), and this is the area we are going to explore now.

A hiatus hernia is very common, especially if you have joined the over-fifties club. Three in ten people over fifty will have a hiatus hernia. Scientists estimate many more will be affected, but with very mild symptoms or none at all. In effect, many of you will never realize you have this condition. There are two types of hiatus hernia: the sliding hiatus hernia and the rolling hiatus hernia.

The treatment for both types of hernia is the same, unless surgery is the only option for a sliding hiatus hernia, so we are not going to separate the discussion of treatment for the two. However, we will

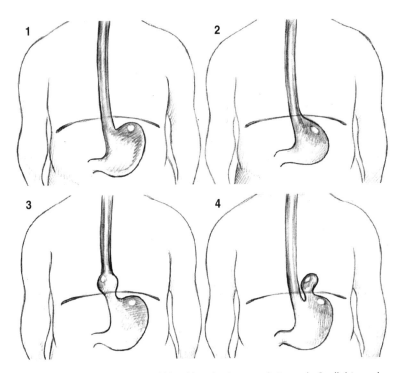

FIGURE 2.1. The four stages of hiatal hernia: 1. normal stomach; 2. slight erosion at top end of stomach; 3. sliding hernia; 4. rolling hernia.

make you aware of the complications of having a hiatus hernia. The continual acid erosion at the lower end of the esophagus can lead to scarring. This scarring contracts and thickens leading to a narrowing, or stricture, of the lower end of the esophagus where food can get stuck. This can cause a condition called Barrett's esophagus, where abnormal cells begin to develop on the inner lining of the esophagus. This condition needs careful observation, as abnormal cell reproduction can lead to cancer of the esophagus.

Sliding Hiatus Hernia

Eight out of ten sufferers have this most common form of hernia. With the sliding hiatus hernia, the junction between the esophagus and the stomach, which contains the gastroesophageal sphincter, slides up through the diaphragm and creates a balloon like structure. Most of the time you probably won't even notice that you have this condition. Because this type of hernia can slide in and out of position (hence its name), the symptoms are likely to be intermittent. According to current medical opinion the most likely symptom you will experience is heartburn, and this is most likely to occur after meals. That said, it is possible to endure heartburn without a hernia, and vice versa. Other symptoms may include:

- Finding swallowing difficult or painful

- Belching

- Chest pains

- Shortness of breath

A sliding hiatus hernia acts as a trap for reflux, so any acidic fluid that remains trapped will come into contact with your esophagus. This means that it can irritate and erode the lining of the esophagus, creating ulcers. (The chapter on ulcers will tell you more about this.)

Rolling Hiatus Hernia

With a rolling hiatus hernia the junction between the esophagus and the stomach that contains the gastroesophageal sphincter stays below the diaphragm as it should, but a portion of the stomach slides up through the diaphragm and lies beside the esophagus. The difficulty with this type of hernia is that the portion of the stomach that gets trapped can lose its blood supply. We call this a strangulated hernia and it often requires an emergency operation. Thankfully, this condition is much less common than the sliding hiatus hernia. Some people have the misfortune of having both types, which is called a mixed hernia.

Hiatus Hernia Syndrome/Vagus Nerve Imbalance (HHS/VNI)

This is the most interesting finding I (AP) have come across in my years of clinical practice, both as a nurse and a nutritional therapist. It answered my prayers for some of my most discouraged clients, and I am really excited to tell you about it. Before I begin let me tell you a little about the vagus nerve. This is one of the most important nerves in the body. It is part of the parasympathetic nervous system, which must always be in balance with the sympathetic nervous system. The sympathetic nervous system provides us with the acute stress response for fight or flight so we can get out of trouble fast, while the parasympathetic nervous system is the calming influence after the stressful event that allows us to come back to earth. The vagus nerve originates in the medulla oblongata at the stem of the brain. The medulla is responsible for involuntary body functions such as regulating breathing, heart rate, blood pressure, and stomach muscle vomiting response. The vagus nerve travels from the medulla down through the neck and chest, through the hiatus and into the stomach. On its way it also branches out to many other areas of the body. The name speaks for itself, in that "vagus" comes from the Latin word for "wandering." In addition to sending messages from the central nervous system to the organs of the body, the vagus nerve also sends messages back to the brain about the state of these organs. About 80 percent of these messages are actually sent directly back to the brain, so it appears to be a kind of master tuner of the body.

So why am I telling you all this and what significance does it have for your hiatus hernia? Well here's the thing: Professor Steven Rochlitz has coined the term hiatus hernia syndrome/vagus nerve imbalance (HHS/VNI).[1] He hypothesizes that by late middle age, 50 to 85 percent of people have this undetected condition, and it may in fact be a predictor of life expectancy for the following reason: Since the vagus nerve runs through the hiatus, it becomes trapped if you have a tightening of the hiatus as you would in the case of hiatus hernia. When the sufferer becomes stressed, his or her body engages the fight or flight mechanism, which shuts down the digestion. This becomes a negative feedback loop, creating havoc within the digestion and causing a secondary effect on other body organs. Imagine the familiar scenario where dominoes are all standing on end so they can just touch each other if they fall over. One domino flicked over leads to a chain reaction until all the dominoes have fallen over. This is the kind of effect we get when the vagus nerve is imbalanced.

Carey Reams, PhD, a renowned biochemist, says something that irritates the nervous system could be the underlying cause of what Rochlitz describes. Vagus nerve imbalance could be due to heavy metal toxicity, a known nervous system irritant. Heavy metals such as mercury, arsenic, and lead have been named. Allergies could also be an issue.

I would also like to add to this the possibility of anyone who had a vagotomy and pyloroplasty surgery in the 1960s and 1970s could fall prey to HHS/VNI. This surgical procedure was a standard treatment for those with gastric ulcers fifty years ago. The vagotomy part of this surgery severed part of the vagus nerve to reduce acid secretion because it was believed (and some still believe this) that high levels of stomach acid caused gastric ulcers. Pyloroplasty was a procedure to widen the pyloric sphincter at the base of the stomach to encourage stomach emptying. This was done because reduced stomach acid means that it takes much longer for proteins to be broken down and food stays in the stomach too long. This can cause a whole host of secondary symptoms. (In a short while I will share a case study that I think demonstrates this well.)

So, back to Rochlitz and his discoveries. He sees a remarkable similarity between hiatus hernia syndrome and angina. Both can cause similar symptoms, and both can occur after the same triggers, such as overeating, exercise, and heavy lifting. From my own experience, those I have seen with atrial fibrillation have all been subject to vagotomy and pyloroplasty surgery or have had GERD for years. We do need some proper studies to substantiate a potential link here (but it won't earn anyone a cent, so I think we will have to live in hope).

It's not only the oldies amongst us that can fall prey to HHS/VNI. Children can too, apparently. Rochlitz tells us that the epidemics of asthma, dyslexia, learning, and behavioral problems in children may in part be the result of HHS/VNI. He says that the wheezing type of asthma that includes chest muscles that seems to "lock" may be one of the most frequent side effects of hiatal hernia. Rochlitz finds that children with dyslexia, attention deficit hyperactivity disorder (ADHD), autism, Asperger's syndrome, asthma, and allergies almost always have HHS/VNI.

The hyperactive child's inability to sit still may be due to the fact that sitting down makes the symptoms of HHS/VNI much worse. Most seats are very unnatural; car seats are the worst of all! Children in this category, according to Rochlitz, almost always have mercury toxicity. This can come from the mother's amalgams during pregnancy or from thimersol in vaccines.

Another condition, called Schatzki ring, can cause the lower esophageal sphincter to become thickened and hardened like scar tissue. The sphincter cannot open and close as it should due to this buildup, and it may be open when it should be closed, causing GERD. Alternatively, it could be closed when it should be open, in which case food can become trapped in the esophagus. This in turn can cause breathing difficulties, anxiety, or heart arrhythmias such as atrial fibrillation. Breads and fibrous meats are the foods most likely to get trapped. This issue happens a lot in the elderly with dementia. People with this condition may need to have regular stretching of the ring via endoscopy. O. Arthur Steinnon, MD, has hypothesized that factors such as progesterone imbalance (which is linked closely to pregnancy) and the imbalance of intestinal hormones such as cholecystokinin (CCK) and secretin may be associated with Schatzki ring. CCK is known to trigger gallbladder contraction and the release of bile into the duodenum in response to the ingestion of fatty foods. [2] Trapped gas exacerbates this condition markedly. A person with the condition may feel like they are dying, as a racing heart, hypertension, and asthma take over, only to be relieved by belching.

The saddest thing about all of this is that the traditional medical community does not recognize HHS/VNI. Hiatus hernia is seen to be minor, and therefore it has no connection to any other condition that might manifest. Most patients suffer with ADHD, Schatzki ring, or other conditions for decades or even a lifetime without resolution. Their hernia remains unnoticed while their allergies get worse. The foods causing the problem cannot be properly detected even with the use of a food diary because with a sliding hiatus hernia they will react to a food one day (when the sphincter is closed and food is trapped in the esophagus—the stomach is "up") and not another (when the sphincter is open and stomach is "down").

Interestingly, personal communication with Dr. Patricia Kane, Director of the Neurolipid Research Foundation and BodyBio.com, has highlighted another factor to consider here. When GERD is at its worst we should also consider the state of the gallbladder (more on this later). If the gallbladder is functioning suboptimally—if it is sluggish due to stone formation, CCK feedback loop failure, parasites, or heavy metals—then bile cannot be released, and the stomach swells in response, causing the "stomach up" feeling). This further exacerbates the GERD symptoms, in particular the heartburn, or that familiar feeling of high bloating. Dr. Kane is saying we should always check the gallbladder first.

SO, WHAT'S EATING YOU?

In view of what I said earlier, I don't think you can really do justice to your hiatus hernia without addressing your stress levels. We don't really like to talk about stress because it has negative connotations. If we succumb to stress we are identifying ourselves as weak or feeble, or even pathetic, or unable to cope with the world as everyone else does. I hate to say it, but this attitude is a figment of our imagination. Stress is everywhere. The pace of life is so fast and the need to achieve is so great that most of us don't even recognize or acknowledge the stress that surrounds us.

Some of us are even addicted to our own adrenaline, the body's hormonal response to stress. We tend to call these people type A personalities: always rushing and on the go, doing many things at once, not enough hours in a day—in other words, "wired." You all know someone like this, and you may even recognize yourself in the description. No worries; the first rule is recognizing and accepting that succumbing to stress isn't feeble or pathetic. It's normal in today's world. Knowing this sets the scene for change.

The other thing to note here is that stress can be both positive and negative at the same time—for example, the excitement of organizing your wedding or your next house move. These are great times, but the stress response is the same as if you had just lost your lifelong spouse. Stress is insidious; we don't notice it creep up and bite us because we are used to the low-grade impact it has on us generally. I discussed the acute stress response earlier, but what happens if this acute response becomes chronic? Well, put it this way: it isn't a pretty sight. Let me give you an example of an elderly client I saw for early stage dementia.

Jim (not his real name) was a seventy-six-year-old retired railway manager with early dementia. Presenting symptoms were obvious forgetfulness (loss of the previous thirty years of memory) and panic attacks (Jim had recently lost his wife, who had been his main caregiver). As his history unfolded it became apparent that he had almost lost his life to a bleeding gastric ulcer at the age of thirty, when he was found collapsed at home. Thankfully, as a known ulcer sufferer Jim was rushed into surgery for a vagotomy and pyloroplasty. His teeth had already been removed five years earlier as a "cause" for his ulcer. Although his initial recovery from surgery was uneventful he never seemed to attain full digestive health. Since his operation he needed to maintain digestive wellness with antacids. This began with products such as milk of magnesia; later graduating to Gaviscon, an over-the-counter digestive aid; and then to prescription proton pump inhibitors (PPIs).

Jim had been a regular known sufferer of the old faithful Helicobacter pylori bug since we started to understand it in the nineties. Interestingly, alongside his gut issues, he also began to suffer with panic attacks. In 1988 Jim was again rushed into hospital, this time with atrial fibrillation. Without going into too much detail, this is an abnormality in heart rhythm where the top two chambers of the heart beat faster than the bottom two chambers. This can lead to blood clotting due to the erratic and inappropriate pumping action of the heart, which can then result in strokes or heart attacks. Pretty serious stuff! All the usual tests were carried out and no cause was found.

Jim was eventually stabilized on a myriad of heart medications including statins, warfarin, ace inhibitors, and digoxin. He still had atrial fibrillation, albeit at a slower rate, and he still had the dreaded panic attacks. What was interesting at this point was that he chose to retire early. He and his wife settled into a routine of regular meals, holidays, and grandchildren. Although he was noted for being a worrier and there always seemed to be an underlying anxiety he managed this well and in fact became quite laid back with his new life. Sadly, his wife died after a long fight with cancer. Overnight the panic attacks resurfaced, worsening by the day to the point where he was convinced he was dying. That was when he came to see me (AP).

I ran a Gastro test to get a measure of whether he had enough stomach acid to digest his food. This showed he was making very little stomach acid. Tests for heavy metal toxicity highlighted mercury (presumably from exposure to coal burning when he was a railway fireman), aluminum (presumably from many years of antacid use), nickel, and lead. He also had high homocysteine levels, indicating an increased need for vitamin B_{12} and folic acid (which was also low on the regular general practitioner (GP) blood tests) as well as betaine (used to replace stomach acid and as a methyl donor to help reduce homocysteine).

My own conclusions in this case (and I can only hypothesize) are:

- underlying low-level anxiety depleted valuable minerals, leaving his body open to initial mercury toxicity from his job, which irritated the vagus nerve.

- His worrying/anxious nature directly predisposed him (via the stress response) to low stomach acid.

- He may have initially had high stomach acid, which caused the stomach ulceration. The surgery to reduce stomach acid and his stressful work lifestyle set up the domino situation.

The end result was that low stomach acid may have resulted in GERD. This in turn possibly had a hand in trapping the vagus nerve (if Rochlitz is correct), thereby precipitating panic attacks. Low stomach acid had preset the mechanism for low B_{12}[3] and folic acid deficiencies, which ultimately allow the rise of the neurotoxin homocysteine in the blood. This correlation has been cited in many papers on heart disease, dementia, and Alzheimer's disease. In fact, the 1995 Framingham Heart Study[4] confirmed the role of homocysteine in the development of both heart disease and dementia. In addition, Jim had the extra burden of heavy metal toxicity, both further irritating the vagus nerve.

The Consequences of Hypochlorhydria (Low Stomach Acid)

Stomach acid (pH) is essential for the digestion of the nutrients in food. It is crucial to have a pH level of around 2 (which is very acidic) in the stomach to ensure adequate secretion of intrinsic factor, a glycoprotein produced in the stomach that is required for vitamin B_{12} absorption. This pH level also helps to sterilize the stomach, killing off any bacteria that enter the body with the food you eat. A proper pH level is important to ensure good protein digestion, as proteins are broken down into the amino acids that are responsible for repairing and rebuilding the tissues of the body. Nutrient release from food also depends on stomach acid and stomach enzymes; for example, vitamin

B_{12} is released from animal foods such as meat and eggs by acid and pepsin.[5]

Folic acid absorption in the small intestine is also influenced by stomach acid.[6] It liberates the minerals calcium, zinc, and iron from food and maintains their soluble forms until they are absorbed in the small intestine. There are also a few studies that have identified that low stomach acid has a bearing on the absorption of the fat-soluble vitamins A and E. With this in mind, we might expect to see more conditions such as pernicious anemia, osteoporosis, poor immune function, and cancers as a result of HHS/VNI low stomach acid: these most certainly occur as part of the aging process. Folate deficiency is associated with blood diseases and cancers.[7] It has been found that administration of folate may assist the methylation pathway, thereby reducing toxic homocysteine. Protein malnutrition has been shown to be a factor in the lowering of immune cells, so ultimately a good dietary approach is crucial.[8]

Esophageal Cancers

Cancer of the mucous membranes in the esophagus is well worth some thought, as it prevents a person from eating completely. Esophageal cancers tend to occur more commonly in men than women by a ratio of 3:1.[9] Adenocarcinoma of the esophagus is one form of esophageal cancer that is believed to be a result of GERD. Studies performed on the incidence and prevalence of adenocarcinoma in certain populations have identified an association between this and a deficiency of the vitamins A, B_6, C, E, and folate.[10] Dietary fiber is said to be protective against the development of adenocarcinoma. If you are unfortunate enough to suffer Barrett's esophagus you will be checked regularly for signs of this, so that's good.

In the United States adenocarcinoma is the most common form of esophageal cancer. Here in the United Kingdom our old friend, the squamous cell cancer of the esophagus, is more common. Smoking and drinking is said to cause most cases of this. However, there are a few other conditions that may predispose you to it, such as achalasia. This is where those peristaltic waves we spoke about earlier are too sluggish to move food along effectively, so swallowing becomes an issue. Lack of trace minerals such as selenium may also play a part, or a work hazard such as being exposed to ionizing radiation, or the good old human papilloma virus (HPV). HPV is more well-known for causing cervical cancers in young women, but it can set up home in any mucous membrane. It is also the troublemaker that brings on the warts. Vitamins A and C have antiviral properties, so a shortfall of these important nutrients could be part of the picture. Achlasia is really not a nice cancer to have because it really limits your food intake due to the obstruction of the esophagus caused by the tumor. This may mean a liquid diet is necessary, which makes life incredibly difficult, as it may be impossible to obtain enough calories and nutrient-dense food to maintain weight and fight the cancer. In some cases a gastrostomy feeding tube may seem to be the only option to prevent starvation. We do have solutions that you may find incredibly useful to get around this problem, however, so please do not despair yet.

The Western medicine approach to esophageal cancer is surgical removal of the sections of the esophagus where the cancer is in its early stages and hasn't yet spread (metastasized) to other organs. This requires pulling the stomach up into the chest cavity and attaching it to the upper esophagus just below the throat. This has its own postsurgical risks, including leakage from the new surgical join and chest and heart problems because there really isn't enough room in the chest for another organ. A compromise has to be made by the body, and scar tissue can build up around the new join, causing a stricture, which then won't open to allow food to pass. If this happens, then the only course of action is a gastrostomy feeding tube, inserted directly into the stomach from the outside of the body. When surgery is not possible, chemotherapy is the treatment of choice in the hope that the tumor will shrink. In many cases it does, and nutritional support may be an adjunct to help you through chemotherapy.

This is not about choosing natural therapies over Western approaches because the two can work together. Most of the time it isn't a personal choice, it's more about what is appropriate for the stage of the cancer at that point in time. Many of our patients undergo chemotherapy to shrink the tumor and in-between treatments they come to us for nutritional support to help them to support their body in dealing with the effects of the chemotherapy. From my own experience with these patients this is by far the approach to aim for; it brings the best of both worlds and lets them be active partners in their own care.

One exciting development in natural therapies for cancer is Gc-MAF (see the Action Plan, Section 1 for more detail). There is a mouthwash version of this therapy that is helpful for tumors in the mouth and throat, and possibly for inflammations in general

One patient I knew was a young man with a small family. He had everything to live for and a three-month death sentence on his head due to adenocarcinoma with metastases. He could hardly swallow, so all of his food had to be liquidized. This meant loads of carbohydrates that were fermenting behind the tumor, causing a frothing in the stomach and lower esophagus. This further impaired his ability to maintain weight and derive a good nutrient base from his diet. Lucky for him he was highly focused. He had all his meals analyzed for calorie content and nutrient status and placed on a spreadsheet for discussion. We don't expect this from all our patients and indeed not from him, but how wonderful it was to have this baseline.

Long-term reflux indicated potential low stomach acid and of course one should never start supplementing stomach acid with a tumor present, so we took the safe option. We asked him to improve his juices with essential oils and soaked nuts/seeds from our Power Drink recipe (more on this later). To ease the load on his digestion we asked him to thin these down and sip them throughout the day rather than have them as a meal or snack. In addition we also asked him to take one tablespoon of apple cider vinegar (ACV) in warm water at the beginning of the meal to acidify the stomach enough to support protein digestion. We also asked him to take carbonate-based electrolytes after the meal to alkalize the small intestine, thereby supporting digestion farther down his digestive tract. Once we improved his carbohydrate/protein/fats intake ratio his "foaming" decreased markedly. However, he was really struggling with what we term high bloating because the apple cider vinegar (being acid) and the electrolyte salts (being alkali) were fermenting in his gut too. High bloating occurs at the upper end of the stomach as opposed to deep inside the intestines. This was the last thing he needed. Allowing more time between the dosing of each was not effective either. Following a bit of head scratching and a bit of background research we looked at the possibility of mixing the two products, letting the fermentation off-gas, then drinking the mix after it had gone flat. I have to say I never expected this to work for him but thankfully it did, and we are all wiser for the experience. He went on to have chemotherapy, supported by oral and occasional intravenous vitamin therapy. After only one round of chemotherapy his tumor has shrunk enough for him to graduate to soups and a small amount of soft food.

While he is nowhere near remission he is now in a much better position in terms of how his body can be supported throughout the rest of his treatment. Sometimes the smallest changes can have dramatic effects, and he is testimony to this. (Please go to the last chapter for treatment options for any of these conditions.)

Helpful Recommendations

In addition to taking things easy and controlling stress, there are some practical things you can start right away to stop or ease your symptoms. Eliminating caffeine and excitotoxins such as monosodium glutamate or aspartame is really important. Perhaps the most nerve damaging substance is mercury. Rochlitz says that perhaps due to its high metabolic rate, the vagus nerve preferentially absorbs mercury. There is no evidence to support his theory, but that doesn't mean we should ignore it. Sparkling drinks such as soda should also be avoided. Most forms of exercise will exacerbate the hernia so you need to be careful which exercises you choose, and start slowly. Food combining may help to reduce or eliminate gas. Ensuring that you don't eat complex animal proteins and carbohydrates together at the same meal will help to take the pressure off the digestion.

CHAPTER 3

ULCERS AND
HELICOBACTER PYLORI

The previous chapter focused on the way food gets into the stomach and the problems that occur there. In this chapter we will be looking at the stomach itself, the route out of it, and the biggest single thing that goes wrong there—ulcers.

Ulcers of the stomach and duodenum are known together as peptic ulcers (it can be difficult to tell the difference between them, and it doesn't matter a great deal anyway). Ulcers used to be a huge part of what doctors did, but while they are still big, their importance is in decline. This is due to two Australian doctors, who in the early 1980s figured out that the main cause of peptic ulcers was a bacterium called *Helicobacter pylori*. (More on this later in the chapter.)

STRUCTURE AND FUNCTION OF THE STOMACH

The stomach looks like a J-shaped balloon, with a sphincter (a ring of muscle that can open and close) at each end. The top sphincter is supposed to prevent food and the stomach contents getting back up the esophagus, and it is in this area, where the digestive tube goes through the diaphragm, that things go wrong in GERD (gastroesophageal reflux disease). At the other, downstream end of the stomach is the pyloric sphincter, which regulates when food leaves the stomach for the duodenum, the first part of the small intestine. There it receives bile from the gallbladder and liver, and bicarbonate

37

(HCO_3) and enzymes from the pancreas, which together start the next phase of digestion.

What was still food when it entered your stomach is completely changed by the time it leaves. The chewing of the food and the churning action of the stomach muscles has broken up its physical structure, and stomach acid has already started to break up its component molecules. At this point the stomach contents are also rather acidic—sufficiently so that people with an eating disorder such as bulimia (bingeing on food and then inducing vomiting) can actually corrode away the surface of their teeth. But the enzymes from the pancreas won't work in such an acid medium, so it needs to be neutralized by the bicarbonate, also produced by the pancreas (more on this in the next chapter).

There are three hormone-driven reflexes that control these functions. Without too much unnecessary detail, this is how they work:

• Gastrin is mainly produced by the downstream end of the stomach (called the antrum), just before the pyloric sphincter, when it senses there is something in the stomach that needs to be digested. It stimulates the upstream end of the stomach to produce acid to do this. This process is also regulated by the vagus nerve, which can be irritated as it passes through the diaphragm (see the chapter on GERD).

• Secretin is produced by the duodenum, the part of the small intestine just after the pyloric sphincter, when it senses there are acidic stomach contents coming through. It causes the pancreas to produce bicarbonate to neutralize the acid, which activates the pancreatic enzymes.

• Cholecystokinin (CCK) is also produced by the duodenum when it senses fats or oils coming through from the stomach. It causes the pancreas to produce and release its digestive enzymes, and the gallbladder to release the bile it has been stockpiling. Both of these are needed to digest fatty foods.

An important component of the whole process of digestion is mucus. This sticky, slightly slimy stuff coats all your internal surfaces-

—the nose, throat, and lungs; the mouth, gullet, stomach, and intestines; the eyes and ears; and the urinary system. That is why all of these are sometimes called mucous membranes. The purpose of mucus is to protect the cells of these surfaces from organisms such as bacteria, viruses, and parasites, and from chemicals such as stomach acid. A healthy adult produces about a liter of mucus every day (more, obviously, if you have a streaming cold, for example).

ULCERS

Ulcers happen when the mucus layer gets broken and acid gets through and damages the surface cells of the stomach or duodenum. Originally we didn't know why or how this happened although we knew that smoking, drinking too much, spicy foods, stress and worry, and certain drugs and diseases could cause it. We thought it was always caused by too much acid being produced. The one thing we could do well was neutralize or block the acid. As the expression says, "If you only have a hammer, everything looks like a nail."

So, doctors prescribed a lot of antacids, alkaline chemicals that neutralized the acid, and later a whole new class of drugs, starting with cimetidine (often known by the brand name, Tagamet) in the late 1970s, that stopped the cells of the stomach wall from producing acid. These drugs worked, more or less, but you had to stay on them for life.

The other solution was to have an operation to cut part of the vagus nerve, thus reducing the stimulus to the stomach to produce acid. The main problem with this option was that in many cases it also removed the stimulus to open the pyloric sphincter and empty the stomach; so another procedure was needed to fix the sphincter in the open position. Not an ideal solution, but it sure kept the surgeons busy.

The diagnosis of ulcers is still big—one American in ten has an ulcer at some time in their life—but it used to be huge. The incidence has been coming down since the 1970s, due firstly to changes in lifestyle—cutting down on smoking and drinking, mostly. Just look at how much Humphrey Bogart smoked and drank onscreen, and remember it was a pretty accurate reflection of his real life habits. He died of cancer of the esophagus at fifty-seven.

When I (DD) was a med student, just new on the wards, I was asked to admit an old gentleman with stomach pains. It turned out he had been admitted with an ulcer back in 1945, at the end of World War II. The army doctors then had told him to "only eat white food," and this was all he had eaten for the next quarter-century—milk products, white bread, cauliflower, white fish. He was skinny, of course, practically starving, and it hadn't worked—he still had the ulcers. In a way he was lucky only to have had the ulcers for twenty-five years because there are three serious complications that can happen:

1. Ulcer hemorrhage, in which you bleed from the ulcer either slowly for a long time or sometimes suddenly, which can quickly be fatal;

2. Ulcer perforation, when the ulcer corrodes all the way through the wall of the gut, the contents leak out into the abdomen, you develop peritonitis, and can go into shock;

3. Cancer, particularly of the stomach.

HELICOBACTER PYLORI

We also thought that no bacteria could survive the acidity of the stomach, which still is almost true. So there was no way that stomach ulcers could be caused by an infection.

Then we figured it all out, in one of the best scientific serendipity stories ever. Way back in 1875 German researchers had seen spiral-shaped organisms (i.e., helical bacteria) under the microscope in samples of human stomach lining. But they couldn't grow the bugs in culture, so the research went nowhere. A whole hundred years later, in 1979, an Australian pathologist, Robin Warren, saw them again. He and another doctor, Barry Marshall, started to research this and try to grow them in the lab. They had no luck until Easter of 1982, when they closed the lab for the five-day Easter holiday. When they came back in to the lab they found their culture plates had grown colonies of the organism. It was originally given the name *Campy-*

lobacter pylori, which was later changed to *Helicobacter pylori* (*H. pylori*).

Warren and Marshall published their work in the *Lancet* in 1984,[1] but it got a skeptical reception at first. To prove the bacteria actually caused stomach disease, Barry Marshall drank a beaker full of the cultured bugs in solution. Several days later he came down with nausea and vomiting. An endoscopy showed that: (a) he had gastritis, an inflammation of the stomach, and (b) the *H. pylori* bug was there. That still didn't prove that the bug caused the disease, but when Warren and Marshall then showed that an antibiotic worked to treat the gastritis, the job was done. In 1994 the U.S. National Institutes of Health (NIH) made it official in a published opinion that *H. pylori* caused most ulcers. Eleven years later, in 2005, Warren and Marshall received the Nobel Prize for Physiology or Medicine for their discovery.

Scientists believe that half the world's population is infected with *H. pylori*. It flourishes in families, especially those living together in close quarters where it is easily transmitted from person to person. It is not unusual to see a whole family infected. That doesn't mean they will all have ulcers or any stomach symptoms at all; 90 percent of people with ulcers have *H. pylori,* but no more than 20 percent of people with *H. pylori* get ulcers—more if they also take nonsteroidal anti-inflammatory drugs (NSAIDs) though. (More on that in the next section.)

The helical (corkscrew) shape of *H. pylori* means it can burrow into the mucus lining of the stomach. This protects the bacteria from stomach acid, but it doesn't protect the cells in your stomach or intestine. Quite the opposite—the presence of the bacteria causes inflammation of the cells lining the stomach or duodenum. This makes them more vulnerable to the natural stomach acid. Additional effects of the *H. pylori* inflammation include the production of more acid in the stomach and less bicarbonate in the pancreas, both of which make the whole situation worse.

H. pylori does not only cause ulcers, it can give you all sorts of symptoms: nausea, vomiting, diarrhea, heartburn, abdominal pains, and even halitosis (bad breath). And in addition to ulcers, it has been linked to more general gastritis, to auto-immune changes in the intestine, and to an uncommon stomach cancer called a MALT lymphoma (MALToma). So it is worth thinking about, and asking your doctor about, if you have any chronic digestive symptoms at all, because if you have it, you probably won't get rid of the symptoms without getting rid of the *H. pylori*. If it's an ulcer that probability becomes a near certainty.

Diagnosis and Treatment of *Helicobacter Pylori*

For a few years back then it was difficult to be sure of a *H. pylori* diagnosis because the tests were unreliable, but they are much better now. With either a stool test or a blood test your doctor can be 95 percent certain that you have or don't have an infection of *H. pylori*. And the "triple therapy" treatment regimens are successful at least 75 percent of the time—more maybe, depending on who you're listening to. So if you test positive for *H. pylori* it probably still makes sense to do the treatment, for most people anyway.

You could argue, of course, that if you have an ulcer you almost certainly have the bug, and so you need the treatment. But the other side of that coin reveals two negative effects of treatment: it kills off the "friendly" bacteria in the large bowel, and it trains the targeted organism to be resistant to the antibiotics. Antibiotic resistance is a well-known problem these days, with Methicillin-resistant *Staphylococcus aureus* (MRSA), the hospital superbug, in so many hospitals. We have been able to watch the bugs learn and get stronger over the years, and this is already happening with *H. pylori*. It's the old adage "What doesn't kill you makes you stronger." The more incomplete or unsuccessful courses of antibiotics are given, the faster the bugs learn resistance to them.

The killing of "friendly" bacteria has been going on for decades, leaving many of us open to infection with fungal organisms such as candida. It may be too late to stop this progression, but we could at least slow it down by treating powerful medications such as antibiotics with respect, and using them only when they are really necessary. We created the mess that we are now in; that's why it's called ecological medicine.

Triple therapy (two antibiotics plus the acid-blocker omeprazole) may be the right thing for you, but there are a couple of things you can do to make it even better. One is adding probiotics; a review of studies in 2006 from China showed that adding a probiotic to a standard triple regimen increased the success rate from 75 percent to 83 percent, and a 2012 study showed that just one week of probiotic, either immediately before or after the triple therapy, will do the same trick.[2] It also halves the risk of the commonest side effect, diarrhea.

The other useful add-on is vitamin supplementation: vitamin C (500 milligrams [mg]) and vitamin E (200 international units [IU]), both twice daily for a month. This pushed the success rate up over 90 percent in a 2009 study.[3] I am not aware that anybody has tried using the vitamins, the probiotics, and the triple therapy all together, but I see no downside to it, so that is my recommendation.

There are a variety of herbal treatments that have an anti-*Helicobacter* effect. Many people in the Arab world swear by Black Seed, *Nigella sativa*,[4] which comes as an oil, and does appear to have a reasonable success rate in getting rid of *H. pylori*. (It is claimed to have a huge range of other benefits as well, of which some at least have been found to be true.)

Jack was an office manager who had a heart attack when he was fifty-eight. He was also receiving treatment for a stomach ulcer at the time. Neither was a surprise, as he was an overweight smoker with a sedentary job who took no exercise apart from strolling down to the pub. But this was just when the smoking ban was starting, so the heart attack gave him the final impetus to give up cigarettes, take up some exercise, and begin a decent diet.

He lost some weight and got fitter by doing this and made a full recovery from the heart attack, but he still had gut symptoms. Originally these had been of the burning, acidic pain variety—which, with the benefit of hindsight we can see were more likely from reflux due to his big fat beer belly than from an ulcer. That problem cleared up when he sorted out his diet and lifestyle, but he was left with a different problem—an intense pain in his abdomen so bad that his colleagues sometimes found him lying flat out on the floor of his office because that eased it a bit.

The regular scans and scopes showed he didn't have a cancer or even an ulcer that they could find. He had been tested for *Helicobacter pylori* a couple of years before with negative results. None of the treatments worked, and it just didn't make sense. Now, there's no such thing as a perfect, 100 percent-reliable lab test, so we rechecked—and got a positive for *H. pylori*. This was also interesting because there appears to be a link between the infection and heart disease.

So he was treated with the standard triple therapy of antibiotics and so on, and the abdominal symptoms went away. Sure, we gave him a probiotic afterward, and he had been on vitamin C and E ever since the heart attack, so they probably helped, but it's three to one that the antibiotic would have fixed it anyway. His case shows that *H. pylori* can cause a whole range of symptoms, not just ulcers.

NSAIDS

Nonsteroidal anti-inflammatory drugs, or NSAIDs, are used every day by millions of people, mostly to reduce the pain of problems like headaches and arthritis. Aspirin is where it all started, and the "pain-relieving" category includes top-selling drugs such as ibuprofen, diclofenac, and celecoxib. And Vioxx—withdrawn in 2004 because it was believed to have killed 30,000 people through heart disease—was an NSAID. It turns out that all of them increase the risk of heart problems, though, and they also give you ulcers.[5]

When you take an aspirin, or any NSAID—and that includes the low-dose aspirin that people take to prevent heart problems—it appears to do a couple of things. Firstly, it interferes with the normal production of mucus, technical name mucin, that coats and protects the lining of the stomach and intestines. That allows the stomach acid, and the aspirin, and any other unpleasant chemicals that may be around, to get to the cells underneath the mucus and damage them.

Secondly, it does what it says on the box: it reduces inflammation, particularly locally, because it will be in much higher concentration there than when it has been spread through the body. The problem is that without inflammation you can't get healing. Inflammation sends out a signal that repair cells and repair molecules are needed, and sets up an increased blood flow to the area so they can be easily delivered. Without the repair cells the cells lining the gut, already damaged by stomach acid and aspirin, cannot repair themselves and just get more damaged. If *H. pylori* is also in the picture, the damage is even worse.

If you have an ulcer and are on NSAIDs, stop them. Now. Find another way to deal with the pain or inflammation—although if you have been on any painkiller for a long time the chances are that what you have now is analgesic withdrawal syndrome. This means that the original source of the pain may be long gone, and the reason you get pain now is the falling level of analgesic in your blood. It's not your fault; the doctors have made you a drug addict. When you do succeed in coming off the painkillers, you will probably find that the pain is no worse than it is now, on the painkillers.

Whatever the cause of your ulcers, once you have removed the cause you need to heal the gut. Go to Action Plan, Section 2 to find out how.

CHAPTER 4

THE LIVER

In one word, what the liver does is homoeostasis—keeping the internal biochemical environment of the body in good working order. Somebody who counted reckons there may be 500 separate processes that the liver does, but they all come down to three main functions: digesting, balancing, and excreting. This also explains the strange anatomy of the liver, which is unlike any other organ in the body.

You can't live long without a functioning liver, so it makes sense to look after it. We hope to show you that it is a plugged-in part of the digestive system, and the source of more digestive problems then we usually imagine.

STRUCTURE AND FUNCTION OF THE LIVER

The portal vein carries blood from the intestines directly to the liver (it isn't really a vein, though, because a vein carries blood toward the heart). All the nutrition that is extracted by the intestines from everything you eat goes in the portal blood to the liver first. So too do a variety of toxins and undesirable molecules that were in the food, the quantities depending on factors such as the leakiness of the gut (see Chapter 8). All drugs and other chemical agents that you swallow follow this route too. Because the liver detoxifies a great number of the chemicals that are delivered to it, including many medications, some only reach the rest of the body in small concentrations, with the larger part being excreted. This is known as first-pass metabolism, and it is an important consideration in drug design.

First-pass metabolism also affects all the other toxins and undesirable molecules that are absorbed from food, particularly if the gut is leaky. The capacity of the liver to filter toxins can get overloaded and the leakier the gut the greater the chance of this. An overloaded liver will allow both normal, inactivated toxins and still-active ones to be excreted in the bile. No more than an hour after eating a meal, the toxins it contained may have been absorbed, gone through the liver, and passed down the bile duct back into the intestines again.[1]

Balancing

Most of the blood supply to the liver comes through the portal vein; only about a quarter comes through the hepatic artery (from the heart). To understand what happens next, we need to look at the microanatomy of the liver. All the hepatocytes, the working cells of the liver, are arranged in tiny lobules—cylinders with a hexagonal cross-section. All the big vessels coming in and out of the liver divide and redivide until there is a branch inside every lobule, so every lobule contains branches of:

- The portal vein (quite large branches, known as sinusoids), bringing blood and food components from the intestines

- The hepatic artery (much smaller), bringing fresh oxygenated blood from the heart

- The hepatic vein, leading away from the liver to the heart

- The bile duct, leading back to the intestines and so out of the body

This setup brings all the nutrients that you eat, and all the molecules circulating in your bloodstream, to the liver cells, which do the homoeostasis: they store and release, they build up and break down many molecules that we need for day-to-day functioning.

Even supposedly healthy food molecules can become too much for the liver to handle (at least carbohydrates can), and then we get fatty liver, also known as NASH (Non-Alcoholic Steato-Hepatitis). "Steato-hepatitis" just means fatty, inflamed liver, so it is also called

NAFLD, Non-Alcoholic Fatty Liver Disease. The alcoholic version is faster and more severe, of course, but NASH is usually associated with obesity and Type II diabetes, which create their own problems. Get the diet right and this is easily fixed.

Excretion

The tiny bile canaliculi in the liver lobules lead eventually to the bile duct. This duct flows out into the duodenum, the part of the intestine immediately after the stomach, but with a diversion into the gallbladder. The liver produces bile at a fairly steady rate, but it is only needed in the intestine when there is food to be digested, so the body stores it in the gallbladder. While it is there it is slowly concentrated. If certain components become super-saturated (too concentrated to all stay dissolved), they can precipitate out and form gallstones. These can sit in the gallbladder for years, but if something causes them to be expelled from the gallbladder they can cause pain, and even jaundice, as they pass down the narrowing bile duct towards the duodenum, until they either pass into it or the surgeons take over.

As well as its excretory function, bile is also necessary for the absorption of dietary fats. The bile salts act like detergents and break up the fat into tiny particles, micelles, that are easily digestible. Along with the fats, we also absorb the fat-soluble vitamins A, D, E, and K, and some other important nutrients. So anything that impairs the flow of bile will interfere with this. You can usually tell it is happening because the dark brown bilirubin and other pigments in bile are what give normal stools or feces their color. Pale stools means lack of bile, poor fat absorption, and probably poor detoxification too.

LIVER DISORDERS

Over 700 liver transplants are performed in the United Kingdom every year. However, the number of deaths from liver disease is over 10,000. There are about 6,000 liver transplants and 31,000 deaths per year in the United States. Most of those will be due to chronic cirrhosis and fatty liver, but there is one nasty poisoning scenario you should know about, which can cause liver failure, described below.

The most obvious symptom of liver disease is jaundice, when first the whites of your eyes, and then your skin, turns yellow. This is due to a build up of bilirubin, a natural product of red blood cells that is supposed to be excreted in the stools. But lots of liver problems don't cause jaundice, and jaundice can also be caused by a blockage of the flow of bile, usually by gallstones (this is dealt with in the next chapter).

Liver Failure

The most common cause of acute liver failure in both the United States and the United Kingdom is acetaminophen poisoning (acetaminophen is also called APAP, or paracetamol in the United Kingdom). There are more deaths from this than from acute hepatitis; it's pretty hard to pin down, but the U.S. Food and Drug Administration reckons there could be as many as 980 deaths a year linked to the many over-the-counter (OTC) medications, such as Tylenol, that contain acetaminophen.[2]

Those are the numbers; now let's put a human face on it. Acetaminophen is a very widely used OTC painkiller and fever treatment, and the majority of people who die from it never intend to. They just take it for their pain, never realizing how toxic it is: just eight of the tablets a day for a few days can cause liver damage, and sixteen taken all at once would kill some people. The United Kingdom reduced the maximum number that can be sold in a pack to sixteen to prevent deaths, but it has made very little difference.

Sometimes people take a whole handful of acetaminophen as a cry for help—a parasuicide. The next day, they may wake up feeling fine and assume that it has done nothing. It isn't until two or three days afterward that they start to get vague abdominal pains, and by the time they seek medical advice it is too late; their liver is already failing. Without a liver transplant they sink into a coma and die.

And yet the liver doesn't just have one mechanism for getting rid of acetaminophen; it has at least three—sulphation, glucuronidation, and (usually a small proportion) oxidation. Unfortunately the oxidation (by CYP450 enzymes) pathway produces a much more toxic molecule called NAPQI. When the other two enzymes get overloaded much more goes through this pathway, and the resulting buildup of NAPQI can rapidly deplete the liver's glutathione, which is central to the whole intracellular antioxidant defense system. Without this defense cells die, and the liver dies.[3]

The treatment for this—the only treatment, apart from a stomach pump if you get it early enough—is N-acetyl cysteine (NAC), a slightly tweaked version of the natural amino acid cysteine. Even this has to be given early enough to block the downward biochemical spiral. If you are hospitalized with liver failure they will give you NAC, probably intravenously (in a drip), but you can buy the oral version yourself.

If it were a vitamin, acetaminophen would have been banned years ago. It is extraordinary that you can still walk into a pharmacy and buy the stuff. Show some respect for your liver and don't take it!

Fatty Liver, NASH, and Cirrhosis

Together, fatty liver, NASH, and cirrhosis form the "final common pathway" to chronic liver damage—in other words, all roads lead here. Well, three main roads do, all of them important to us in the twenty-first century Western world. They are:

- Alcohol excess

- Metabolic syndrome

- Infectious hepatitis

Very roughly, each of these three accounts for almost one-third of cases of liver damage, and there are some far less common causes such as drug damage and malnutrition.

Without getting too bogged down in precise detail, these are the three stages to the process leading to liver failure:

Stage 1: Fatty liver
A buildup of fat, mostly triglycerides, throughout the liver. This is the first sign of liver damage although a blood test may show some raised liver enzymes. If left untreated this will progress to the next stage of disease in one-third of cases.

Stage 2: NASH

Non-Alcoholic Steato-Hepatitis: fatty liver plus inflammation. Of course, if alcohol is the factor, or even just a factor, change this to ALD (alcoholic liver disease), and CUT IT OUT!

Stage 3: Cirrhosis

Fatty liver, plus inflammation and scarring (fibrosis), and cell deaths. This soon becomes irreversible, and the liver progressively fails in its task of homoeostasis. Levels of toxic metabolites build up, and essential ones like albumin (protein) and clotting factors fall. Eventually the sufferer will sink into a toxic coma (hepatic encephalopathy).

Treatment

Liver disease is one disease complex for which medicines have very little to offer and surgery even less. The only real treatments are nutritional. Now, you might think that in a disease called fatty liver the dietary treatment would be to avoid fats, but in reality the opposite is true. The fats that build up in the liver are triglycerides, which are derived from sugar and carbohydrates in the diet much more than from fats. And one of the key problems in metabolic syndrome is resistance to insulin, which transports sugars, not fats, into cells. That, and the obesity that goes with it, have only been major problems since we started refining sugar and invented junk foods.

So the core of treatment for fatty liver (stage one) is the low-carbohydrate high-fat ketogenic diet. (See Action Plan, Section 1 for further details.) When overweight people with fatty livers were put on this diet for six months their liver health improved and they lost an average of twenty-eight pounds.[4]

When the problem is more advanced (stages two and three) people typically lose interest in food and become malnourished, which makes the problem worse. Lots of good food in a basic healthy diet (see Action Plan, Section 1) is obviously needed, but large quantities of some specific nutrients are also valuable. Possibly the most important one is zinc, in which patients with cirrhosis are typically deficient; supplementation helps a lot of the symptoms, including the hepatic encephalopathy.

HEPATITIS

The word simply means inflammation of the liver, and the experience is no fun. The pattern can be acute or chronic, and the cause is basically from infection or poisoning, plus a small number of cases that are autoimmune.

Acute hepatitis is one of the two main causes of jaundice, along with gallstones. Usually the first sign of acute hepatitis is losing your appetite, then nausea and vomiting, with fatigue and pain in the area of the liver. Urine becomes dark brown, and if there are any stools they become pale. If the inflammation is bad enough you may need hospital admission, with an intravenous drip to put back the lost fluids. If things get even worse you may go into liver failure and the coma of hepatic encephalopathy.

For most people, though, it is a much less severe disease—some people don't even turn yellow. The whole thing lasts between ten days and ten weeks and then it is gone, although sometimes acute hepatitis leads to chronic hepatitis.

Chronic hepatitis can last a lifetime, and the symptoms can be pretty vague: ill-health and fatigue, often coming and going (relapsing and remitting, in medical speak) unpredictably. The most serious consequence is the long-term risk of developing cirrhosis or liver cancer.

Infectious hepatitis is nearly always caused by viruses. We used to think there was only one type of infectious hepatitis, but now we know about hepatitis A, B, C, D, and E. They are all in different families of viruses (in other words, they are not related closely at all), they infect you by different means, and they cause quite different patterns of disease.

Hepatitis A

Hepatitis A is usually transmitted by the fecal-oral route, so it is most common in tropical areas where sanitation and hygiene are a problem. Most people in these regions get the infection as a child, which makes them immune to the disease for life. There are actually more adult cases in the United States than in developing countries because we don't catch the illness as children.

When you contract hepatitis A you develop jaundice and feel quite unwell for a while, and may even need hospital care, but then it goes away. It is rare to develop chronic hepatitis after a hepatitis A infection.

Hepatitis B

Unless hepatitis B is transmitted at birth, it is caught from sexual contact or needles. If you have sex with an infected person you have a 30 percent chance of catching it; if you use intravenous drugs you have a 50 percent chance. And, of course, a load of unlucky people caught it from blood transfusions (especially hemophiliacs, who get lots of them) before we started screening donors. Some also even caught human immunodeficiency virus (HIV) this way.

The acute illness can be mild and brief, or more severe and lead to liver failure. If you recover from it, though, you have a 5 percent chance of developing chronic hepatitis.

Hepatitis C

Hepatitis C has the same pattern of transmission as hepatitis B—via sexual contact or needles—we can't be as sure of the numbers for this disease because most people (more than 75 percent) never knew that they had the acute infection, and so did not do anything about it. It is the main cause of chronic hepatitis, with about 80 percent of infected people developing the chronic form.

Hepatitis D

You can only get an active hepatitis D infection if you already have hepatitis B. As with hepatitis B and C, the usual routes are sexual contact or needles.

Hepatitis E

With hepatitis E we are back to fecal-oral transmission, as with hepatitis A. It is usually a mild disease and is described as self-limiting, meaning it usually goes away without treatment. It is only in pregnant women and their babies that it can be more serious, causing a high rate of deaths. If this has anything to do with you, don't read on, see a doctor immediately.

Treatment

You cannot handle acute hepatitis on your own—you need a doctor to do blood tests, monitor your condition, and give you treatments, in a drip if necessary. But that doesn't mean you can do nothing to help yourself.

People with acute hepatitis are usually not that interested in food, but you do need to drink plenty of fluids to support your kidneys, which are handling a lot of the dark brown bilirubin and other molecules that need to be excreted. You also need to give your liver a rest, so definitely no alcohol, no tobacco, no acetaminophen/paracetamol, and no iron supplements, as all of these can make the damage to liver cells worse. The diet should be light and not overloaded with either carbs or fats. There is no particular type of fat that you should be avoiding in your diet—you do need them all.

In the acute phase of any infection you probably need to give the organ a rest, and that is certainly true of hepatitis. All the vitamins and other supplements recommended below for chronic hepatitis may also be useful in the acute scenario. Don't think you can manage it all by yourself, however. If your liver is ill enough to make your eyes yellow with jaundice, then the same thing is happening in your brain, and your judgment is blown by poisoning. You are in no state to judge what you need—you need help!

Chronic hepatitis is a different matter. Drug treatments are less effective and, because you take them for much longer, can be more toxic. You can definitely help yourself in this case.

1. Clean up
You can't avoid the virus, but you can avoid "poisons" that will make the damage worse. The same avoidances apply here as for acute liver disease: no alcohol, no tobacco, no acetaminophen/paracetamol, and no iron supplements—they can all make liver damage worse.

2. Protect

It is easy to think that nutritional therapy is all about giving antioxidants blindly, whatever the ailment. This is not true, but in chronic hepatitis supplementation with antioxidants is definitely justified. Most important of these is N-acetyl cysteine (NAC) and that should be your starting point.[5] Other antioxidants will work synergistically with NAC, so add vitamin C and vitamin E, and optionally vitamin B_{12}, and alpha-lipoic acid.

3. Nourish

In the chronic phase of hepatitis you can start to feed the liver what it needs to repair itself, and lipids (fats and oils) are the most important nutrients here. You will need all of them.

- omega-6 mostly from vegetables

- omega-3 from fish (but not fish oil unless we specify)

- omega-9 is almost entirely oleic acid from olive oil

- saturated fats from animal products and from coconut oil and/or cocoa butter (there you go—a medicinal use for chocolate!)

When dealing with hepatitis we have special requirements, so we need to add two more:

- Butyrate is a very small (short-chain) fat that prevents the damage caused by toxins (it *inhibits toxin-induced aberrant lipid metabolism*).[6]

- Phosphatidylcholine is the form that oils need to be in to be incorporated into cell membranes. Your body makes this all the time, but taking it by mouth (when necessary we use injections too) speeds up the process and helps to get rid of toxic damage.

See Action Plan, Section 1 for much more detail on lipid supplementation using the Power Drink or Neurolipid Cocktail.

CHAPTER 5

THE BILIARY TREE

This chapter is for those of you who have conditions associated with the gallbladder or any of its associated tributaries. As with the other chapters we will give you an overview of the anatomy and physiology, or structure and function of this organ system, followed by the conditions that are associated with its malfunction. Hopefully you have read the chapter on the liver because these two systems are inextricably linked. Anything affecting the liver affects the gallbladder, and vice versa. And any condition that affects the liver and/or gallbladder can affect any other organ in the body. You will see how and why when you read on.

Between April 2005 and April 2006 there were 49,077 gallbladder removals (medical term: cholecystectomy) in the United Kingdom, according to the National Health Service Institute for Innovation and Improvement.[1] In fact, it is such a common operation that most healthcare trusts now have what we call a "care pathway" in place. This is a standard procedure for how the whole process of care is managed for a gallbladder removal from the patient's first visit to the hospital as an outpatient to his or her complete recovery after the gallbladder removal. While we need to appreciate that in an emergency situation this may be your only option, there are steps you can take to ensure that you keep your gallbladder, assuming you have not yet reached the point of no return.

STRUCTURE AND FUNCTION
OF THE GALLBLADDER

The gallbladder is a small sack about 7–10 centimeters (cm) (2.75–4 inches [in]) long and somewhat pear shaped. At its broadest end it is probably about 3 cm (1.5 in) across. So, as you can see, it isn't a huge structure, but it is a very important one all the same. It can hold between 30–50 milliliters (ml) (1–1.6 ounces [oz]) of bile at one time, and it lies on the underside of the liver, attached to the liver by connective tissue. The gallbladder sack is muscular so that when it is triggered it releases bile. Like the esophagus it has an inner mucous membrane that secretes mucus to protect this tiny organ from irritation caused by the concentrated bile salts it stores. It also has an outer serous (watery) membrane to keep it moist so it doesn't stick to other organs or structures. The muscular layer lies between the mucous layer and the serous layer.

As you will know from reading the previous chapter, bile is made in the liver. It enters the gallbladder via two ducts called the cystic duct and the hepatic duct. Once in the gallbladder the bile becomes concentrated five- to tenfold. When partially digested food leaves the stomach and travels into the duodenum (the first part of the small intestine) as chyme, a hormone called cholecystokinin is released by the small intestine, which signals the gallbladder to contract. This contraction releases bile to emulsify the fats in your food, enabling them to be mixed with water and assimilated by the body. Bile is released into the common bile duct, where it flows into the duodenum, meeting the acidic chyme as it leaves the stomach. You can think of bile as a kind of detergent, making the fat globules smaller so the body can assimilate what it needs to keep everything running smoothly. If bile cannot be ejected from the gallbladder for some reason, you can become jaundiced over time.

What Is Bile, and Why Is It So Important?

The main components of bile are bile salts, salt pigments, phospholipids, bilirubin, and cholesterol. Bile salts are the most essential part of bile. They are formed in the liver from cholesterol, so while you might be busy trying to get your cholesterol levels down, think of life without bile. My feeling is that the gallbladder and bile are just not given enough consideration in the medical literature. The general feeling is that we can live without the gallbladder, which of course is true. We hope that when you have read this chapter you will be giving due consideration as to whether you would want to.

There is an emerging new thought assigned to bile acids, which we would like to alert you to in this chapter. They are now thought to be very closely involved as mediators of what we call metabolic disorders, or disorders in which the body is unable to derive energy from the foods we eat. Obesity, type 2 diabetes, high triglycerides, atherosclerosis, nonalcoholic liver disease, and skin and digestive complaints come into (but not exclusively) this category.

In order to make bile we need vitamin C, taurine, oxygen, vitamin B_3, choline, and betaine or trimethylglycine. Once food flows into the duodenum, bile is released to deal with fat and fat-soluble nutrient absorption. The fat-soluble nutrients include vitamins A, D, E, and K, and coenzyme Q_{10}. Once it has done its job, 90 percent of it is reabsorbed back to the liver via the small intestine and reused. These nutrients are very interesting in their own right, as they all have distinct properties. Vitamin A is antiviral and is known to support all the mucous membranes of the body. It is really important for assisting with immunity in both the lungs and the digestive tract. It is also very important for the retina of the eyes and the skin. It regulates skin cell turnover. With inadequate vitamin A we may be prey to viral chest infections, vision difficulties, and what we call lack of mucosal tolerance (food intolerance). Vitamin D has hundreds of research papers linking it to many diseases of the immune system. It helps us absorb and utilize calcium for bone building and again is important for mucosal tolerance. Vitamins A and D are known as the "sunshine vitamins." Vitamin E is a fat-soluble antioxidant that helps prevent fats and oils going rancid. It helps thin the blood, ensuring good circulation. It has to be taken in its natural form as mixed tocopherols and tocotrienols for the best results. Vitamin K controls blood clotting; in the NHS it is the antidote to warfarin overdose. It is also important for immune support and as a bone-building nutrient.

Coenzyme Q_{10} (CoQ$_{10}$) is slightly different than other vitamins in that the body makes its own when we are young. After forty we lose the ability, so we often have to supplement. CoQ$_{10}$ is the spark plug in our mitochondria, the little powerhouses of the cells that make energy. If you take statins you really must take CoQ$_{10}$.

Another factor to consider is that bile is said to help peristalsis. If you remember in Chapter 2, we said that peristalsis is the wavelike action of the longitudinal and circular muscles of the long tube we call the esophagus. It is also active in the rest of the digestive tract, moving food along and preventing constipation and the recycling of toxic waste from the large intestine. Stool transit time from mouth to anus should be less than twenty-four hours to prevent symptoms of foggy head, headaches, or confusion. In the elderly we always associate these particular symptoms with slow transit time.

Taking a supplement to promote bile acids has been shown to reverse fat accumulation by activating hormones that influence weight.[2] Bile acids have also been shown to affect glucose metabolism in type 2 diabetics who were prescribed cholestyramine to thin their bile. Improving bile flow decreased insulin resistance in addition to enhancing insulin signaling in fat cells. The end result was a reduced risk for "diabesity" (a new term for diabetes linked to obesity). Interestingly, bile salts are also bacteriostatic; that is, they can stop bacteria from reproducing. They cannot kill bacteria already in residence, but keeping the digestive system "clean" by preventing more is really useful. They work with the immune system to remove harmful bacteria from the small intestine before it has a chance to take a hold. The last thing you need if you have digestive problems is SIBO (small intestinal bacterial overgrowth), which we will talk about later. Another study has found that bile also has anti-inflammatory effects by modifying lipid metabolism. It has been shown to prevent blood clotting in the kidneys, so it could be a useful therapy in kidney diseases, especially for diabetic neuropathy. The antiaging effects of bile acids have also been studied in relation to the management of cell generation and division or growth. Adverse aging has been linked to altered immune function and increased inflammation from a declining ability to digest and absorb foods. In one

Hungarian study, taking bile salts had a significant positive result on the condition of skin in patients with psoriasis.[3]

Now that you can see how important it is to ensure good bile flow, let's take a look at some of the ways bile flow might be disrupted and what the effects of this might be.

There is a point to make here in that people who have celiac disease (we will discuss this in detail later) develop inflammation in the small intestine when they eat gluten. The hormone cholecystokinin (CCK) is made in the first part of the small intestine, so those with

Aged sixty-two, she presented with a long history: a previous cancer and a multitude of other seemingly unrelated health issues: frozen shoulder, right-side migraine, irritable bowel syndrome (IBS), hypercholesterolemia (high levels of cholesterol in the blood), skin rashes, incessant tiredness, panic attacks. The radiation therapy she underwent was successful in eradicating her cancer, but it seriously reduced her thyroid function. When she came to me (DD) she was following a vegan diet to reduce her cholesterol.

Over the course of the next few months it became apparent that most of her health issues were occurring along the gallbladder meridian despite the fact that she had undergone a cholecystectomy three years previously. Despite being armed with all the information on risks and imponderables she was eager to try a gallbladder flush. There are a number of gallbladder flushes on the Internet, but the one chosen was designed by Andreas Moritz.[4] This flush requires a period of fasting prior to relaxation of the biliary tree with Epsom salts, followed by stimulation of the gallbladder with a drink containing olive oil and red grapefruit juice before retiring. The following morning any gallstones should be passed into the toilet.

Her first flush resulted in gallstone excretion for a total of four days, and her second flush gave her relief from all these seemingly unrelated symptoms and improved her liver enzymes.

It was a tough call to make with this lady, and I won't say I wasn't a little panicked myself until I heard from her again.

celiac disease will likely have an impaired CCK feedback loop. The gluten also seems to impair gallbladder contraction, so celiac patients have what we call a very low bile ejection fraction. A hepatobiliary (HIDA) scan would be needed to confirm this.

Biliary Parasites

This is really a topic you probably would rather not hear about. After all, who wants to think that we have parasites living inside us, creating havoc? The truth is that these little critters do live with us but they are generally balanced by beneficial bacteria, so they don't really cause us any harm. You will be hearing more about this later, so we will just give you the nuts and bolts for now. When our immune system is not as good as it should be, or we are run down after illness or stressful events, these guys can get a bit too happy and run wild. Roundworm and trematodes (both worms classified under the term "biliary fluke") have been identified as potential disrupters of bile flow.[5] The parasite may be acting as a nest for gallstone formation as the body constructs a cholesterol outer layer around the fluke to protect it from the symptoms of worm infestation. The end result can manifest as cholecystitis or cholangitis, both of which are inflammations of the gallbladder.

Generally speaking, roundworm (*Ascaris*) infection is said to be prevalent only in countries with poor standards of public health. If you or a member of your family have been visiting one of these countries then it's well worth ruling these parasites out as a cause for sluggish bile output. This cause of acute biliary symptoms is second only to gallstones, and an estimated 25 percent of us worldwide are said to be infected. Many of us will never know we are infected. Anyway, if you have these little pests in your biliary tree you will certainly have them in your intestines, so that should make it fairly easy to determine with a fecal smear. If you have a severe case you are likely to be suffering with intermittent right upper quadrant abdominal pain, vomiting, and possibly fever. Continuous upper quadrant pain really requires more investigation.

What about trematodes? These are flat leaflike little pests, varying in length from a few millimeters (mm) (considerably less than an inch) to many centimeters (many inches). They are a lot more trouble than biliary flukes because they are long-lived and can cause progressive damage to the host (you). If you eat a lot of raw fish or sushi then you need to protect yourself from this guy. It is hermaphroditic (contains both male and female in the same organism), so it can reproduce more easily. The larvae are released into the duodenum where it can migrate up the biliary tree to set up home. This can result in thickening of the bile duct wall and may ultimately result in bile duct obstruction. The gallbladder may then become enlarged and in some cases may become diseased and necrotic (the tissue dies and starts to rot). At this point surgical removal will be the only option. If this condition is left unnoticed or untreated it can set the scene for cholangiocarcinoma (cancers of the biliary tree). So far we are unsure of the exact mechanism involved with this change, so we need to concentrate our energies on prevention for now. We will discuss more about this treatment later.

Gallstones

It is probably safe to say that anyone reading this will have heard of gallstones, and that's because they are really common. About 20 percent of women and 8 percent of men over forty have them, and that's an interesting fact in itself. By the time you get the symptoms of gallstones you probably have had them for about eight years. You see, once they begin to form they grow at a rate of 2.6 mm per year. Approximately 85 percent of gallstones are said to be "mixed," meaning that they contain a mix of cholesterol, bile salts, bile pigments, and organic salts such as calcium salts. The other 20 percent are called "pigmented" stones, which are composed mainly of minerals or metals such as aluminum. Stones that are pure cholesterol or pure pigment (calcium bilirubinate) are extremely rare.

We used to have a saying in Western medicine that the majority of gallstones occur in the "fair, fat, forty, female, and fertile" group. The "female" bit is probably because of increased cholesterol synthesis or suppression of bile acids by estrogen, which is considered to be the female hormone. We live in a world of potential estrogen dominance caused by xenoestrogens, chemicals that mimic and increase the production of estrogen in humans. These include oral contraceptive use, hormone replacement therapies, hormone-disrupting pesticides and preservatives in food, and overuse of plasticizers and phthalates that can leach out of our plastic bottles and food containers, especially when they are heated or holding fatty or oily foods. These xenoestrogens also occur in consumer goods such as cosmetics, shampoos, oil-based coatings, and, of course, our old favorite, bisphenol A (BPA). This substance is considered the most serious of all in terms of hormone-disrupting chemicals. All this has a major effect on female health, but we have seen gallstones in young teenage men who have a tendency toward obesity. Typically they also show outward signs of estrogen dominance, such as "man boobs."

It isn't only external xenoestrogens such as those mentioned above that disrupt hormones in this way. We can do a lot for prevention by eating sensibly; by balancing the amount of proteins, carbohydrates, and fats we eat at each meal, and not forgetting a good supply of our old friend, dietary fiber. Fiber will help the body to remove excess hormones through the digestive tract and out in the stool.

A diet high in refined foods such as white bread, pasta, confectionery, and cakes leads to elevations in blood glucose levels. These foods are broken down too quickly during digestion resulting in the glucose spike, and the body responds by secreting the insulin hormone to correct it. Insulin is known to block the rise of progesterone in the second phase of the female menstrual cycle, and too much can lead to potential estrogen dominance.

A high intake of refined sugars is also a risk factor for gallstones as well as bile duct cancers because the sugars will increase levels of blood lipids. Rapid weight loss can also be a risk factor for developing gallstones. During active calorie reduction the concentration of cholesterol in bile initially increases. Secretion of all bile acids is reduced during weight loss, but bile acids decrease more than cholesterol until everything rebalances again. If you are following a weight-loss program losing more than one pound per week and you have elevated triglycerides you should make sure that you follow a regime to maintain bile solubility. Gastrointestinal diseases such as Crohn's and celiac disease and cystic fibrosis are also known to increase the risk of gallstones. Normally 90 percent of bile acids are reabsorbed in the small intestine, but when you have a condition involving inflammation of the small intestine the cells of the gut are unable to reabsorb bile acids. This reduces the bile acid reserve and the rate of bile excretion. Triglyceride-lowering drugs such as those containing fibric acid (fibrates) can also increase your risk, as these drugs reduce triglyceride in the bloodstream by increasing its excretion via bile and digestion. Food intolerances or allergies can be another factor to consider with gallstones. If you have known food allergies you might want to read another book in this series, called *The Vitamin Cure for Allergies*.

So, How Would You Know If You Have Gallstones?

One of the most prominent symptoms is what we call biliary colic. This is an intense pain in the center of your abdomen (belly) just below the breastbone and above the naval. It can also occur in the upper right of your abdomen, with the pain radiating up into the right shoulder. You can also get pain right between the shoulder blades. The intensity of the pain is quite alarming, and it can last anywhere from a few minutes to an hour. Visiting the toilet, passing wind, or being sick will not relieve the pain. This is because there is usually a stone lodged in the common bile duct, and it needs to be passed for the pain to subside. Luckily this doesn't happen very often, but it can make you feel sickly or give you a hot flush. (Menopausal ladies will know how this feels so don't confuse it, girls.) You will find that the colic occurs generally after a fatty meal. If the pain doesn't subside, you develop a temperature, or you become jaundiced, then you must visit your doctor in case you have developed a condition associated with gallstones called cholecystitis.

While cholecystitis is not a medical emergency, it does require treatment to prevent it from leading to complications. One of these complications is gangrenous cholecystitis, which can cause a serious infection that could keep you in the hospital for a while. The gallbladder could also perforate, spilling its contents into the abdominal cavity, resulting in a more serious peritonitis. *That* is a medical emergency.

Cholangitis

You may not have heard of this condition because it too is associated with gallstones. It is a bacterial infection in the common bile duct and it generally occurs when a blockage such as a stone is present or when bile flow is sluggish. Even before you have gallstones the bile in the gallbladder can resemble sand or river sludge. This makes for a sluggish flow, creating a nice home and the opportunity for bacteria, parasites, worms, and yeasts to populate the area. (You can compare this to a compost heap if your stomach is up to that challenge.) Treatment of gallstones, parasites, and tumors may prevent a recurrence for some; others may require a stent procedure to keep the bile duct open.

Bile Duct Cancer

There does not seem to be a consensus on the possible causes of bile duct cancers, but some risk factors have been considered and we are getting a clearer idea of its origin. Research indicates that those who suffer with inflammatory bowel conditions such as Crohn's disease are at increased risk. People who are born with genetic malformations of the bile duct, such as choledochal cysts, also have a higher risk. In areas of Asia and East Africa cases are thought to be caused by the liver fluke. It's those dreaded worms again! Whatever the cause, cancer of the bile duct is the mother of all evil diseases. Once it blocks the bile duct the flow of bile from the liver to the intestine is impaired, causing backflow into the tissues of the body. This is when you start to turn yellow, especially in the whites of your eyes and in your skin. Bilirubin cannot be excreted in the bile any longer, so your stool becomes paler. Instead it is excreted in the urine, making the urine look really concentrated and dark. Measuring bilirubin in the urine tells us that the bile duct is blocked. By this time you are looking pretty yellow.

Diagnosing and Monitoring Bile Duct Cancer

There are a number of tests that can be used to diagnose bile duct cancer. One of these is an ultrasound scan, the type you get to ensure all is well with your baby when you are pregnant. Sound waves bouncing off the biliary tree area build up a picture on the screen. Ultrasound can detect abnormal patterns or structures within the biliary tree. It is a painless test, but you do have to fast for six hours beforehand.

You may also have a computed tomography (CT) scan. If a tumor is found you will get used to CT scans because they are used to monitor the progress of treatment in cancer patients. The CT scanner takes a series of pictures in slices that build up a three-dimensional picture of the area. Again, this is quick and painless. You may be asked to drink a radioisotope so the tumor can be seen more easily. If you have asthma or an allergy to iodine you should tell the doctor so that this step can be missed out for you. A spiral CT spins around the outside of your body taking pictures in a spiral motion to make cross-sectional pictures.

A magnetic resonance imaging (MRI) scan is the next possibility. There are many more MRI scans undertaken now than there was in the past as most hospitals have their own scanners. You lie inside the MRI scanner, which is really noisy, but you will likely be offered headphones playing music to make the test a little more bearable. Sometimes a white dye is injected into your arm before the scan. This helps to pick up more detail in the image.

Another test that may be used is an endoscopic retrograde cholangiopancreatography (ERCP). This is a more invasive test and you will be given a sedative before it is carried out. This is a type of x-ray you can see on a television screen. You will need to fast for six hours before the test, but the good thing is that this test can also be used to unblock the biliary tree if necessary. An endoscopy tube will be passed down your throat into your stomach and duodenum. The doctor can look down the microscope tube to see the duodenum from the inside. He can also pass an ultrasound probe down the endoscopy tube to show more detail.

Angiograms may be used, which like the ERCP require fasting. A catheter is passed into the large vessels that surround the biliary tree to see if the cancer is affecting blood supply to the area. A dye is injected into the catheter and is followed on screen as it circulates within the arteries. To be sure of the diagnosis it will be necessary to take a sample of cells (biopsy) from the tumor site to send to the laboratory for histology.

Finally; a laparotomy may be the only test left if the appropriate test from the list above delivers inconclusive results or if it is thought none of them would be helpful. In this case a small incision is made in the abdomen under general anesthetic. The surgeon inserts a laparoscope to look for evidence of cancer. If the cancer is still localized the surgeon may be able to remove it, or at least unblock the ducts.

Cholecystokinin (CCK) Feedback Loop Failure (Hormones)

CCK is an amazingly interesting area for anyone who has chronic fatty acid deficiency. How do you know if you do have this? Well, for a start, your skin will be dry and flaky or you might have a chronic condition such as autistic spectrum disorder, psoriasis, or even mental health issues. You might even have a condition that has its foundations within the field of hormone disruption/imbalance. Some of these include:

- Premenstrual syndrome
- Menopause
- Cancer
- Accelerated aging
- Hair loss
- Fatigue
- Osteoporosis
- Weakened immune system
- Cognitive impairment
- SIBO
- Decreased libido
- Skin problems
- Allergies
- Appetite loss
- Anxiety
- Sleep disorders
- Depression

We are not saying that all of these are caused solely by fatty acid deficiency, but it certainly would be a large part of the picture. "Hey, hang on!" we hear you say. "I eat my three portions of oily fish a week, and I'm snacking on nuts and seeds. I'm even eating some saturated fat because you said that was really important." We have to say this is very unusual because we have been fed media hype for years saying fats are bad for us. Most of us are fat phobic. Well, as the saying goes, it isn't what you eat—it's what you digest and absorb. Of the patients we have seen with any of these conditions there has always been at least a modicum of impaired digestion. It isn't until the right questions are asked that the answers reveal themselves. We wouldn't expect you to connect the two, especially if you come for help with your psoriasis, hair loss, or osteoporosis.

"What the heck have these conditions got to do with digestion?" "Doesn't everyone get wind (flatulence)?" "I don't get constipated; I go to the bathroom every three days." These are classic comments received when we pry into patient's toileting habits. We hate to say it, but, no, these aren't normal. What is normal is a nice quiet digestive system that empties itself cleanly and painlessly one to two times daily. If you don't have this, then you have something that needs fixing— and you can bet it will be somewhere within this CCK feedback loop.

Let Me Tell You about This Feedback Loop

You have read by now that the food bolus you have chewed well (hopefully) and swallowed has travelled down the esophagus; remember your friend from the earlier chapter on GERD? Once it is in the stomach you will remember that the proteins in it are denatured, or broken down by the action of stomach acid and pepsin inside the stomach. Once it becomes an acid soup (chyme) the pyloric sphincter in the bottom of the stomach releases it into the duodenum.

The arrival of the chyme in the duodenum triggers two hormones, cholecystokinin and secretin. A hormone is your body's chemical messenger service. Glands of the endocrine system make them, and they travel to other sites via the bloodstream where they affect other body tissues or organs. They are so powerful that only a minute amount is needed for dramatic effects anywhere in the body. So back to CCK and secretin. CCK, literally translated from the Greek, means "to move the bile sack." It stimulates the release of bile from the gallbladder and the release of digestive enzymes from the pancreas. It also acts as a hunger suppressant. Secretin, on the other hand, is responsible for regulating the acid level (pH) of the duodenum by inhibiting stomach acid and ensuring the release of bicarbonate from the pancreas. It also maintains osmotic pressure in the rest of the body via its action on the hypothalamus, pituitary, and kidneys. The pH level of the stomach should be 1 to 3 (highly acidic), and the pH of the duodenum should be 6 to 7 (slightly alkaline). You can now see that bicarbonate release is crucial since digestive enzymes are meant to work in an alkaline environment. Any deviation from this has the potential to create a dysbiosis (more on this later) that may then disrupt hormones and neurotransmitters or set up inflammatory reactions anywhere in the body.

So, back to hormones. These really important chemical messengers are made from fats and proteins. Can you see the problem here? With an inability to digest and absorb fats due to a sluggish gallbladder, gallstones, or the inability to produce bile in the liver, we can't make CCK. Without CCK we can't trigger the gallbladder or pancreas to release their respective digestive aids.

If you recognize this description, then we're guessing you have a lot going on that you were unaware had CCK feedback loop failure as an underlying cause. We aren't painting a gloomy picture without offering a solution, so don't despair. Depending on your age, you may need to provide support to all digestive organs that are dependent on the CCK feedback loop in order to bypass or eliminate the need for this mechanism for a long time; maybe for your lifetime. However, the results may be well worthwhile in terms of symptom resolution and health gains.

Treatment of Complicated Biliary Tree Issues and CCK Feedback Loop Failure

Many of you will need the support of a professional to initiate your program, but you will soon get the hang of managing your own health and the rewards it will bring will make it worthwhile. To try and put CCK feedback loop failure into a clinical perspective, let me (DD) tell you about another case of mine.

This patient is a female intensive care nurse, aged fifty-six. Her family history offers some key points: her father has a history of gastric ulcers/GERD, atrial fibrillation, and vascular dementia. Her mother had Hashimoto's hypothyroidism, depression, and lung cancer.

She presented with psoriasis, social anxiety/shyness, premenstrual syndrome replaced by menopausal symptoms, multiple food allergies, hair loss, low immunity, candida since her late teens, chronic fatigue for ten years, and celiac disease diagnosed five years ago, but possibly lifelong.

The patient was born by emergency caesarean section (C-section) and was not breast-fed. She had amoebic dysentery at the age of three months, which was said to be from a Malaysian parasite her father caught while in the army. Her psoriasis started a year after she started school, hair thinning around eleven to twelve years of age, thrush/candida and premenstrual syndrome (PMS) around sixteen to seventeen years of age. She also had ten amalgam fillings placed during her childhood. Food allergies, biliary colic, and chronic fatigue commenced with her first pregnancy at age twenty-eight. Interestingly, this child was later diagnosed with autism spectrum disorder.

So how did I analyze this case? First, I considered her antecedents (predisposing factors): two parents with possible dysbiosis (Hashimoto's is an autoimmune condition that may originate from an imbalance of gut bacteria, said to give rise to autoantibodies that attack the thyroid itself). That said, hypothyroidism reduces metabolic rate and this can have a negative impact on digestion such as constipation, flatulence, bloating, and reduction in digestive secretions.

Next, I looked at triggers (factors that may ensure that a condition will manifest): caesarean birth and lack of breast-feeding. Caesarian birth means the baby misses out on obtaining valuable commensal gut flora and beneficial bacteria while traveling down the vaginal canal during birth.[6] According to Anita Kozyrskyj, babies who had been born by C-section had lower levels of *Shigella* bacteria and *Bacteroides* that are thought to be the first colonizers of the gastrointestinal (GI) tract. In addition she found higher levels of *Chlostridium difficile* in babies who were bottle fed. Other researchers, including the researchers Guaraldi and Salvatori, have since supported this.[7]

Then I considered mediators (factors that keep the condition going): her diet of refined foods, with her low stomach acid preventing adequate protein absorption; a diet low in essential fatty acids, in other words, no oily fish, nuts, or seeds; CCK feedback loop dysfunction that may have occurred as a result of the original Malaysian parasite.

What did her tests show? Her gastro test confirmed low stomach acid. A positive Murphy's sign (Murphy's sign is a form of palpation of the gallbladder while you are lying on your back. If Murphy's sign is positive you will feel pain on inhalation. You can see a doctor performing Murphy's sign here: https://www.youtube.com/watch?v=NMce3WJeIyU) confirmed a sluggish gallbladder (suggested by an earlier mineral analysis of her hair). Stool testing confirmed the presence of *Candida parapsilosis* and *Candida albicans* yeasts, mold, *Klebsiella pneumonia* and *pseudomonas* bacterium, and the *Blastocystis Hominis* parasite. Mitochondrial profiles confirmed heavy metals (nickel) blocking energy production (indicated by low levels of zinc, manganese, and magnesium). Lymphocyte sensitivity testing confirmed mercury, silver, and nickel (from her amalgam fillings) as being problematic.

So, all told, her genetic predisposition may have set her up with a dysbiosis, further exacerbated with the Malaysian parasite. She wasn't protected by her own immune system due to her caesarean birth and from being bottle-fed. Various stressful challenges such as starting school, adolescence, and pregnancy, not to mention an adrenaline-focused job, further exacerbated her dysbiosis and ultimately her symptoms. It is unclear whether this lady may have suffered with celiac disease for many years or if it developed during her first pregnancy. However, malabsorption is a key symptom, leading to mineral deficiencies such as zinc, selenium, and magnesium. These minerals are suppressed by the presence of mercury and nickel. Regarding her CCK feedback loop failure, it could have been caused by parasites heading up the biliary tree causing sluggish bile flow. It could equally have been due to heavy metal toxicity or continual stress, reducing her ability to make stomach acid. Mercury has a great affinity for the gallbladder and nickel is well known to cause skin diseases such as contact dermatitis, which is not unlike psoriasis in appearance.

I used a staged approach to resolve some of this lady's issues. It was important to first support her digestive system to ensure good digestion and absorption. This was achieved with high-strength betaine hydrochloride (HCL) to replace stomach acid. Then we worked on gallbladder support, by adding a combination of Beta Plus, Beta TCP (a commercial preparation of the beta form of tricalcium phosphate [TCP]), taurine, ox bile, and beetroot complex, iodine, and Super Phosphozyme, orthophosphoric acid with vitamin C and calcium, with enteric-coated peppermint when she had colic. Digestive enzymes and potassium bicarbonate were taken after meals and probiotics specific to small intestinal bacterial overgrowth (SIBO), including *Lactobacillus plantarum, Lactobacillus rhamnosus,* and *Lactobacillus salivaricus,* plus *Lactobacillus rhamnosus GG.* She followed a modified neurolipidketo diet (more on this later).

Once her digestion had calmed and she felt somewhat better, the heavy metals were chelated with methionine and zinc (for the nickel), selenium, chlorella, and magnesium (for mercury). Then we implemented the 5R approach (described in Action Plan, Section 1) to improve her digestive health further.

So we hope we have demonstrated the importance of good bile flow in order to keep the digestive system clean of parasites and opportunistic bacteria. Hormones, peristalsis, and youthfulness are dependent on adequate bile flow and fatty acid synthesis. Today's Westernized diet and lifestyle have a massive impact on whether your bile is flowing and keeping you young and healthy. The gallbladder and CCK feedback loop are central to good digestion, detoxification, and elimination. Please do not ignore yours.

CHAPTER 6

THE PANCREAS

The pancreas: it's hard to find, easy to forget, but you can't do without one. It is hard to find because it is usually tucked in behind the stomach and the bowel; if the doctor presses high up on your abdomen when examining you, what he is usually feeling is the stomach—unless the pancreas is inflamed, when it can certainly cause you pain.

STRUCTURE AND FUNCTION OF THE PANCREAS

The shape of the pancreas is pretty similar to that of a crayfish or prawn without its head, running most of the way across your abdomen. All this tissue produces the pancreatic juices that are the next phase in breaking down and absorbing the nutrients in the food you eat. These flow through a duct that runs along the whole length of the pancreas and comes out into the duodenum, the part of the intestine immediately after the stomach. The common bile duct, carrying bile from the liver and gallbladder, routes through the pancreas and comes out through this same opening. If a stone exits from the gallbladder, comes down the bile duct, and gets stuck at this common exit point, it will also block pancreatic secretions from getting into the intestine. Likewise, inflammation of or damage to the pancreas that blocks the bile duct can prevent it from draining normally.

Hidden inside the pancreas are also some small clumps of cells called the islets of Langerhans. They manufacture and release insulin, which is necessary to transport sugars into cells. This is what malfunctions with Type I diabetics, who are likely to become reliant on daily injections of insulin. Type II diabetes is different. It occurs when cells become so full of fat molecules that insulin has less and less effect on them, and they become insulin resistant. Diabetes is dealt with in another book in this series, so we won't describe it in depth here. You can see that it has a lot to do with being overweight and therefore with what you eat, but remember that this fat is caused much more from sugars and carbohydrates in the diet than from fat in the diet.

Pancreatic Enzymes and Other Secretions

The pancreas produces digestive enzymes and bicarbonate (HCO_3), both of which are necessary for the digestion of food. As mentioned earlier, the stomach produces a lot of acid that starts to break down the particles and molecules of food that you swallow; when this mixture moves out of the stomach and into the first part of the small intestine, the duodenum, it is very acid. The pancreatic enzymes only work in an alkaline environment, however, so the acidity must be neutralized by the release of the alkaline HCO_3.

When the body detects that there is stomach acid in the duodenum it triggers a hormone called secretin. This hormone causes a solution of HCO_3 and water to be made by the pancreas and released into the duodenum. When it detects that there is fat and/or protein in the duodenum a second hormone called cholecystokinin (CCK) causes the pancreatic enzymes to be released. The name cholecystokinin translates literally (from the Greek) as "gallbladder mover," and CCK performs that function too: it causes the gallbladder to contract and release its stored bile through the same exit point into the duodenum. If all goes well, there is a large and sophisticated set of digestive factors released onto the food all at once.

The pancreas produces fifteen different digestive enzymes that fall into three categories:

- Amylases, which break down starch

- Proteases, which break down protein

- Lipases, which break down fats

Digestion of Fat

It seems the body has the digestion of all the food components nicely covered, but this is only partly true because the digestion of fats lags behind that of starch and protein. In the acidic environment of the stomach the breakdown of the latter two goes well, but very little digestion of fats actually occurs. It is not until the pancreatic lipase enzymes get to work that the breakdown of fats really progresses. A further step is then necessary before we can effectively absorb the fats in our diet. The bile that is secreted in response to food (same time, same place, and same trigger as pancreatic juices) contains molecules called bile salts. These cause the fats in our diet to form into nanoparticles called micelles, which can then be absorbed by the cells in the wall of the gut.

All this is rather complicated, but that is the point. Because it is so complicated, when things go wrong with the digestion of nutrients in our food, they generally go wrong with fat digestion first.

PANCREATIC DISORDERS

There are really only three things that can go wrong with the pancreas: it can underfunction, known as exocrine pancreatic insufficiency (EPI); it can become inflamed, known as either acute or chronic pancreatitis; and it can develop cancer.

Pancreatic Insufficiency

It is only recently that medicine in general has recognized the disorder of pancreatic insufficiency.[1] It is like a closely related disorder, celiac syndrome, in that doctors tend to think that it's binary—either you have the full-scale disorder, or you don't have it at all. But that's not really true for either disorder. For every person with a major problem there are a lot with a minor version.

Also, the whole process of digestion is a chain reaction. Each step triggers the next one; for example, when the stomach contents move into the duodenum, they set off the hormones that activate the pancreas and gallbladder. If something goes wrong with the production of stomach acid, for example, it may in turn fail to activate the pancreas. In fact, it only takes one thing to go wrong somewhere between the lips and the pancreas itself to disrupt this carefully coordinated process.

Causes and Triggers

Chronic inflammation caused by infections (such as *Helicobacter* in the stomach), by immune reactions to food (as with celiac syndrome), or due to unexplained reasons (such as Crohn's disease of the bowel) can set off the problem, as can small intestine bacterial overgrowth (SIBO), described in more detail in Chapter 7. Surgery on the digestive tract, for whatever reason, can obviously alter its complex interactions and cause the pancreas to malfunction. This is even true of gastric band surgery for weight reduction. There is a fifty-fifty chance of experiencing nausea and sometimes vomiting after this procedure, in which case the digestive process is inevitably disrupted, and so is pancreatic function.

Symptoms

If your pancreas malfunctions severely and acutely, you will need to be in the hospital. That's not what happens in EPI, in which it creeps up on you gradually and may be masked by other problems in the digestion. In fact there may be no obvious symptoms at all, but the two most common are flatulence/gas and fatigue.

Flatulence. Flatulence happens when gas builds up in the intestine. If food is not digested properly, as happens with EPI, it cannot be absorbed and it stays in the digestive tract. Bacteria get to work on it and produce hydrogen and methane gases. A limited amount of this always happens in the large bowel; everybody farts, after all. If the digestion goes wrong, however, the wind may start in the small intestine, giving an unpleasant feeling of distension or bloating. The pressure of this gas flattens out the tiny villi in the small intestine, making malabsorption worse by reducing the surface area available for the absorption of nutrients.

One way to tell where the problem that is causing the bloating lies is by its timing. If abdominal bloating happens while you are eating or within fifteen minutes, it is almost certainly due to a stomach issue because the food hasn't gotten any farther. If it happens more than thirty minutes after finishing a meal it is almost certainly due to a pancreatic issue.

Fatigue. In severe cases of EPI there are a number of specific deficiency diseases that can occur (see below), but lesser degrees of the problem are more likely to cause general fatigue, a lack of energy, and feeling rundown. There can be weight loss too, but often people eat more to compensate, so the weight loss is masked.

Malabsorption of Fat and Other Nutrients

The extra complexity of the way we digest fats means that it is often the first bit to go wrong in EPI, which can cause the following symptoms:

- Steatorrhea; oily, smelly (and sometimes pale) stools because of their high content of undigested fat

- Muscular weakness and fatigue due to malabsorption of fat-soluble vitamin D

- Osteopenia and possibly osteoporosis due to malabsorption of fat-soluble vitamin D

- Night blindness and dry eyes due to malabsorption of fat-soluble vitamin A

- Abnormal bleeding, showing as bruising under the skin, or blood in the stools or urine, due to malabsorption of fat-soluble vitamin K

  Other malabsorption disorders that can occur include:

- Edema (usually around the ankles) due to lack of protein

- Anemia due to lack of iron and/or B vitamins

- Muscular cramps and spasms due to lack of magnesium

- Peripheral neuropathy (pins and needles and/or loss of sensation in fingers and toes) due to lack of vitamin B_1

Treatment

The first thing to do for patients suffering with EPI is to replace what the pancreas presumably is not efficiently producing: the HCO_3 and/or the digestive enzymes. See Action Plan, Section 2 for full instructions on how to supplement or improve your diet to accomplish this. The second is to clean up your diet, removing all the foods likely to be overloading or irritating your pancreas. See Action Plan, Section 1 for how to do that.

Pancreatitis

Pancreatitis comes in two versions: acute and chronic. We're not going to tell you how to treat acute pancreatitis because you can't; it's too dangerous. *You absolutely need to be in a hospital, and possibly in an intensive care unit.* In any case, the symptoms—pain, tenderness, fever, loss of appetite—could be something else just as serious, like a burst appendix. Go see a doctor!

Symptoms

Pancreatitis happens when the pancreatic enzymes, intended to digest your food, end up digesting the pancreas itself. This is known as autodigestion. The two commonest causes, each causing about 40 percent of cases, are gallstones and alcohol. The main symptoms are pain, tenderness, swelling, fever, and loss of appetite. The pain is usually dull and constant, located in the upper half of the abdomen, and often spreads through to the back. It feels like something is boring through you, and it gets steadily worse. Your abdomen typically feels overfull and even distended, you certainly lose your appetite, and may vomit and/or have diarrhea.

What can happen in the acute version is that the pancreas, or parts of it, die (called necrosis), the inflammation involves the whole body, you go into shock, other vital organs like the kidneys fail, and you have a one-in-three chance of dying. Don't take that chance.

Chronic pancreatitis is different. The pain may not get very bad, and people often do not bother their doctors enough to get diagnosed.

The pancreas gradually builds up scar tissue (fibrosis) and loses its functionality. This leads to pancreatic insufficiency (described above), and sometimes to diabetes.

Causes

Gallstones can cause pancreatitis because if they are the right size they can get stuck at the common outlet of the bile duct and pancreatic duct and cause back pressure in both. Eventually this pressure can burst through the wall of the duct into the tissues of the pancreas. The "right size" means fairly small because bigger stones tend to get stuck farther up in the bile duct and give you simple obstructive jaundice without damaging the pancreas.

Alcohol does it because it simultaneously overstimulates and inflames the pancreas, and the large quantities of pancreatic juice produced in response can seep through the inflamed wall of the duct into the tissues of the organ.

It is no surprise that a number of other toxins can also trigger or contribute to this disease.[2] The most obvious one is smoking (which often goes together with heavy alcohol consumption); it causes severe oxidative stress, also known as free radical damage. (See any cosmetics advertisement for information about this!) You could describe smoking as an extreme form of environmental pollution, and it is probable that all other forms of environmental pollution can have the same effect. They certainly cause oxidative stress throughout the body, which we can pick up in tests on blood cells, but it's difficult to get tissue samples from the pancreas to prove that it happens there. Experiments on unfortunate laboratory rodents don't really transfer too well to the human condition.

There is also an important interaction between alcohol and the body's detoxification mechanisms, which means that alcohol can make its own toxicity and the toxic effect of other things like smoking much worse. This process involves an enzyme in the liver known as Cytochrome P450 2E1 (CYP2E1), which is one of the phase I detoxification enzymes. This is a complicated area of chemistry, but what these enzymes mostly do is make toxic chemicals more reactive, so that in phase II of the detoxification process they will react more strongly with a neutralizing agent and be excreted still bound to it. So between phase I and phase II the chemicals are more reactive and more dangerous. CYP2E1 does this to alcohol, but also to several other dangerous but commonplace chemicals, such as the pain killer acetaminophen, nitrosamines used to preserve food, certain petro-chemicals, and vinyl chloride from solvents, varnishes, paints, and similar chemicals.

Sustained heavy drinking induces (switches on) the gene for this enzyme, causing the body to produce more enzyme so it can process more alcohol and other toxins. As a result, all of them become more toxic. At the beginning, this happens mainly in the liver and is a con-tributing factor to fatty liver (NASH), as discussed in an earlier chap-ter. But NASH makes the enzyme even more active, and sooner or later enzyme production starts happening in the pancreas as well, and then you have chronic inflammation—pancreatitis. So if you drink heavily and smoke it's a dangerous cocktail for the whole digestion, and decorating the house or working with paints or varnishes could make it even worse.[3]

Pancreatitis has also been reported in people with celiac disease. Nobody seems to know how often this occurs, but it may explain some of the 20 to 30 percent of chronic pancreatitis for which a cause is never identified. We do know that wheat can cause chronic inflam-mation in the gut if the right triggering events happen, and those events include wheat intolerance as well as celiac. In this case it is clear what you need to do about it.

Treatment

Please remember that this advice only refers to chronic pancreatitis because we will not support you in handling acute pancreatitis. All the following would apply if you had the time in the acute form, but you still need your doctors.

Avoidance. "When you find yourself in a hole, the first thing to do is stop digging"—an appropriate saying in this situation. If you are diagnosed with chronic pancreatitis you are likely to be told to stop drinking and/or smoking, and you should heed this advice because they are major factors. If that is hard for you then you are entitled to the assistance of experts in addiction.

Also, cut wheat out of your diet (see later in this book for advice on this). Pancreatitis is a serious enough disease to justify this, and there could be other benefits for your gut from cutting out wheat.

In the past doctors often recommended a low-fat diet because pancreatitis can lead to pancreatic insufficiency. This affects absorption of fats more than that of protein or carbohydrates, so steatorrhea (pale greasy stools) can be a symptom. Just treating that symptom can lead to more serious nutritional deficiencies of fats, however. We should be supplementing them, not restricting them further.

In acute pancreatitis this can be solved by jejunal feeding: putting a tube down the throat, through the stomach, and past the pancreas, giving fats through it and bypassing the triggers such as CCK that activate the pancreas. In the chronic form the solution lies with medium-chain triglycerides, usually obtained from coconuts. These can be absorbed in the small intestine without the need for pancreatic enzymes.

Digestive enzymes. There are two reasons to give digestive enzymes in chronic pancreatitis. Firstly, it is very unlikely that your diseased, damaged pancreas is producing enough enzymes itself, so you do have exocrine pancreatic insufficiency. You need the extra help in digesting your food.

Secondly, the CCK that is produced when food hits the duodenum causes the pancreas to produce more enzymes, which can feed the whole inflammatory cycle. Giving the enzymes by mouth damps down the production of CCK because the body gets the message that there is enough enzyme there already.[4] That's negative feedback for a positive result.

Surgery. There are all sorts of complications that can occur with pancreatitis, and you may need surgery to repair them. They include cysts, abscesses, fistulas, and stenosis (plain old blockage) of the pancreatic duct.

Antioxidants and melatonin. There is a lot of evidence now that antioxidants are helpful in pancreatitis. The problem is that you should have taken them a long time ago because they are much better at prevention than cure. This is certainly true for one of the major naturally-occurring antioxidants, melatonin. Produced at night, it helps us to sleep; as anyone who has taken it for jetlag or on a long-haul flight will know, it helps you sleep but doesn't *make* you sleep (knock you out). At the same time, it encourages healing and damps down inflammation. But melatonin only works well if you take it before the problem starts. With a serious inflammatory process such as pancreatitis, that pushes it down the priority list.

There is another reason why taking supplements of melatonin is not the solution. It will trigger CCK, the hormone that activates pancreatic enzyme production in the duodenum. We were never meant to take melatonin by mouth. We used to think that it was only produced by the pituitary, the gland just under the middle of the brain that regulates all the hormones. In fact, much more melatonin is manufactured in and around the tissues of the gut. Even here it is made mainly in the early night, and it does send signals to the brain, but it is also a major player in healing and repair of the gut.[5] And its production can be disrupted by stimulants that interfere with the sleep/wake cycle (alcohol and tobacco for a start) and by free radicals (also alcohol and tobacco). But stress, excitement, pain, and bright light (including television) can disrupt it too. So, the message is: Get a good night's sleep. It will make a real difference to your healing ability.

To do that you want to avoid alcohol, tobacco, and caffeine completely, and television, computer screens, and all bright lights for a couple of hours before you want to sleep. That should give you melatonin where and when you need it.

There are a couple of natural agents that show promise in helping to treat pancreatitis. One is a herbal extract from the spice turmeric (curcumin), and the other is alpha-lipoic acid, a not-quite vitamin that we can make for ourselves, but sometimes need a booster.

CHAPTER 7

DYSBIOSIS

The small intestine is a long tube about 2.5 centimeters (cm) (less than an inch [in]) in diameter and about 6 meters (m) (about 20 feet [ft]) long. Makes you wonder how we get such a large organ in such a small space, doesn't it? The fact that it consists of a network of coiled loops makes this possible.

STRUCTURE AND FUNCTION OF THE SMALL INTESTINE

The small intestine is composed of three sections.

The duodenum, the first part of the intestines, originates at the pyloric sphincter. As we described earlier, this sphincter is where food leaves the stomach as acid chyme. It is at that point bicarbonate is released from the pancreas to neutralize the acid. Bile from the gallbladder helps too, and the three combined enable further breakdown and assimilation of foods to produce energy and fuel. The duodenum is the shortest section of the small intestine, measuring 25 cm (9.8 in) or twelve fingerbreadths, as its name implies.

The next section of the small intestine is the jejunum, 2.5 m (8.2 ft) long, and then the ileum, 3.5 m (11.5 ft) long. These names probably will not really mean anything to you unless you have had surgery resulting in an ileostomy or you have a feeding tube into the jejunum.

The walls of the small intestine are very intricate. They contain many circular folds, a bit like a soft version of the piped chocolate frosting on a decorated cake. From these folds hairlike structures called villi extend about 1 millimeter (.04 inch) into the intestine. They have the appearance of velvet and are capable of movement similar to plants in the ocean. On these villi are even more tiny cells (microvilli) that make up the aptly named brush border. There are roughly 1,700 microvilli to each cell in the brush border, and they have multiple functions. Significantly, they massively increase the surface area of the small intestine, making this organ the main site of digestion. Digestive enzymes are also produced in the small intestine to enable breakdown and digestion of food. Mucus-secreting goblet cells are also found in large numbers on the villi and in the spaces between villi, called crypts. Cell division is rapid in this organ, due to the incredible amount of work the digestive tract has to do. Cells are replaced approximately every four days compared to a month in other parts of the body. That's an incredible turnover!

We hope you now have a picture in your mind as to what the brush border looks like. This incredible surface area is really important to allow the small intestine to absorb as many nutrients as possible. Interestingly, if we could open up the intestine and flatten it out we could cover a football field with it, so that's worth thinking about. Glucose (from carbohydrates such as fruit, vegetables, and grains), amino acids (from the breakdown of proteins), fatty acids and glycerides (from fat digestion), and cholesterol are all absorbed through the brush border.

When digestion is impaired we start to see the manifestation of all types of disease. We will discuss some of the important everyday diseases, but, before we do, it is important to consider the immune system first. This part of the gut is where our immunity is built. Hippocrates, the father of medicine, wasn't wrong when he said, "bad digestion is the root of all evil."

If you are unable to fully digest fats and oils, large, greasy, and foul smelling stools (often called steatorrhea) result. You won't get a soul to stand downwind of you if you have this! You may feel nauseated after eating fats and oils. If you have carbohydrate/sugar malabsorption you will likely suffer flatulence, bloating, and possibly diarrhea.

This is really unpleasant because the bloating diminishes your appetite significantly, causes inflammation, gives you the cramps, and generally makes for a miserable existence. This is because the microbial balance of the gut becomes disturbed. (We do live with beneficial bacteria, or rather they live with us; normally they are our "partners," so embrace them instead of grimacing.

An old saying states that "Death begins in the colon." Louis Kuhne, a nineteenth century naturopath, and Élie Metchnikoff, a Nobel laureate in the early twentieth century, were two of the first to identify gut bacteria as factors that determine our health. They talked a great deal about intestinal toxicity and we still talk about this today, but today we generally call this inflammation. Once you get to the stage of intestinal inflammation the tight junctions between the cells of the intestine can separate. Protein particles from foods may pass through these junctions, setting up an immune reaction. We will discuss this later in the leaky gut section, so let's get back to our dear friends the beneficial bacteria.

Beneficial Bacteria

What do we mean by the term "beneficial bacteria"? Well, Metchnikoff's belief stemmed from the fact that inside the small intestine we have billions of bacteria residing in our gut. In fact, we are currently aware of about 400 different strains. We won't bore you with all their names here—what is important is that bacteria of the *Lactobacillus* species help keep house for us. They have distinct functions:

1. Development of a competent intestinal and systemic immune system

2. Maintenance of the integrity of the tight junctions between intestinal cells

3. Competition with potential disease-causing bacteria for space and resources

4. Digestion of complex plant sugars (polysaccharides)

5. Absorption of simple sugars (monosaccharides) and triglyceride storage

6. Synthesis of certain vitamins, including vitamin K, B_{12}, biotin, folic acid, and pantothenate (vitamin B_5)

7. Metabolism (chemically changing, using, and excreting) steroid hormones, bile acids, drugs, and dietary carcinogens

8. Production of butyrate as a food source for the cells of the intestines

There are other commonly residing bacteria in addition to these guys, namely *Streptococcus, Enterococcus,* and *Bacteroides.* When all these bacteria are in balance we have a symbiotic relationship with them; in essence, they keep us well. However, genetic predisposition, antibiotic use, poor dietary choices, stress, poor immunity, allergies, and intolerances can all upset this balance, giving rise to a condition we call dysbiosis. This is when the wrong (pathogenic or disease-causing) bacteria overcrowd our beneficial bacteria. In the small intestine we call this small intestinal bacterial overgrowth, or SIBO. In cases of SIBO the walls of the intestine may become inflamed and the tight junctions may widen, allowing partially digested or undigested food particles through. This confuses the immune system and food intolerances rear their ugly heads. We won't be covering this in detail here, so you may wish to consult another book in the series called *The Vitamin Cure for Allergies.* However, we will cover celiac disease because this condition appears to be prominent in many and diverse cases. The lactulose-mannitol challenge test is a good test to find out if your tight junctions are working optimally.

Let's look at some of the factors associated with the balance of this gut microflora.

Age

The gut is sterile prior to birth. The first introduction to beneficial flora is during birth, when the fetus is expelled down the vagina to the outside world. The gut flora begins to resemble that of an adult at around two years of age. As you can probably see here, children born via caesarean section develop a completely different gut microflora, there being a delay in the acquisition of beneficial bacteria.[1]

SIBO is also very common in the elderly and may be associated with malabsorption.[2]

Microbes

Although the exact mechanism is unclear, what we do know is that we can manipulate the balance of bacteria in the gut to effectively create wellness or illness. A specific probiotic bacteria called *Saccharomyces boulardii* given in capsule form has demonstrated a significant reduction in the incidence of antibiotic induced diarrhea.[3]

Diet

The gut microbiome, or ecosystem, is seen as a complex system of interaction with the outside world. It is in constant interaction with the foods we eat, and they will influence the balance of microflora. Infant-feeding regimes can have a profound effect, with bottle-fed babies developing the gut flora more appropriate for an adult. There are hundreds of studies that have looked at specific foods that have a positive effect on the microbial balance. As a result we now have a list of foods we call prebiotics because they feed the beneficial bacteria in our system, thereby encouraging optimal balance. We will give you a list of these foods in the diet section of this book. Other studies have looked at the use of sulfur-containing foods, vegetarian and vegan diets, and isoflavone-rich diets (from flaxseed and soy). While the sulfur foods had a negative impact, the vegan and isoflavone diets had a positive effect.

Drugs

The obvious drugs to mention in regard to upsetting the delicate ecobalance of our gut are antibiotics. By now everyone has heard that antibiotics wipe out all gut flora, good or bad. The term antibiotic literally means "against life." We don't want you to think we are against all drugs, but we have had many years of overprescribing, and prescribing, for viral infections such as heavy colds when in fact antibiotics are useless for viruses. We are not blaming our doctors because we as patients have the mind-set and the expectation that a pill will cure all, and we make that pretty plain when we visit doctors.

And these drugs can save lives, so in some cases they are to be embraced. That said, antibiotics are the drugs most likely to upset the gut microflora; so far from helping your immune system they actually damage it over time.

Other drugs that may have a negative effect on microbial balance are proton pump inhibitors (PPIs). Earlier in this book we said this was the most common prescription patients receive. These drugs reduce the amount of stomach acid and therefore reduce the pH of the stomach and small intestine. This in turn reduces the number of beneficial bacteria in these parts of the digestive system, leaving us open to the invasion of the likes of *Helicobacter pylori, Clostridium difficile,* yeasts, and parasites. The evidence regarding this is still quite sparse so we make no claims here,[4] but this is worth considering.

Drugs that affect transit time in the gut may also affect microbial balance. You may have done the school science test where you ate sweet corn and counted the number of hours before it exited the other end. Well, that's transit time. Drugs like morphine and loperamide (an antidiarrheal drug) have been shown to slow down the gut significantly. Others, such as erythromycin, increase transit time. In both cases the balance of bacteria has been changed in favor of potential disease-causing bacterial populations.

Stress

Nothing you change in terms of your nutrition will have a massive impact if you don't address stress. We talked about the impact of stress in reducing stomach acid, aggravating hiatal hernias, and initiating gastroesophageal reflux disease (GERD). Down at the end of the gastrointestinal tract the result can be anything from simple constipation to irritable bowel syndrome (IBS) to exploding diarrhea. None of these would be a pleasure. The reason for these things happening is, in part, that the poor microflora are so susceptible to stress. A study on monkeys showed that, if the babies were separated from their mothers, they actually shed *Lactobacillus* bacteria out in the stool from the first day of separation. This led to an increased risk of infection.

Stress is also known to reduce the levels of secretory immunoglobulin A (SIgA); this little guy plays a huge part in giving us our immunity in the areas of the body where we have mucous membranes. That includes the whole of the digestive tract, ear, nose, and throat, lungs, urinary, and reproductive systems in both men and women. Low levels of this beneficial bacteria can render us susceptible to all manner of opportunistic invasion by parasites, yeast, or disease-causing bacteria with a catastrophic decline in general health.

SIBO–When Things Go Wrong

We have now talked about the structure and function of the small intestine. We have also briefly talked about the bacteria that reside in there and what their overall functions are. We can now see how important they are, so we sincerely hope the grimace has gone and is replaced by a smile. We are probably going to wipe the smile off now because we need to talk more about bowels. We British have a stiff upper lip about this topic. It's something we hate discussing, and when the topic crops up it's distasteful or unpleasant, like discussing some burglar has broken onto our home and ransacked our personal items. We can stop beating around the bush now, and talk about SIBO.

SIBO, as you recall, is short for "small intestinal bacterial overgrowth." What the phrase means is that abnormally large numbers of bacteria—at least 100,000 bacteria per milliliter (ml) or .03 ounce (oz) of fluid—are present in the small intestine, and these resemble the bacteria of the large intestine or colon more than those of the small intestine. This can set you up with an awful array of symptoms. Check these out:

- Bloating
- Abdominal discomfort
- Diarrhea
- Abdominal pain
- Belching
- Flatulence
- Anemia

- B_{12} deficiency
- Malnutrition
- Reduced bile acids
- Steatorrhea
- Weight loss
- Food allergies
- Brain fog

- Systemic inflammation
- Autonomic dysfunction
- Chronic fatigue
- Restless leg syndrome
- Micronutrient deficiencies such as vitamins B_{12}, A, D, E, B_1, B_3, and iron

That's a whole lot of digestive misery. This needs to be checked out against IBS, nonresponsive celiac disease, and fructose/lactose malabsorption so you have the right condition to work with.

Factors that might lead to SIBO include low stomach acid, a history of PPI use, poor gut motility, collagen vascular disease, immune deficiency, surgery to any part of the gastrointestinal (GI) tract, advancing age, chronic pancreatitis, chronic antibiotic use, low SIgA levels, celiac disease, Crohn's disease, short bowel syndrome, NASH (nonalcoholic liver disease), cirrhosis, fibromyalgia, and rosacea. You can get the tests for some of these from your general practitioner as a starting point and work from there. The other alternative is to have a hydrogen breath test. The test measures hydrogen (H_2) and methane (CH_4) in the breath. Twenty parts per million is the threshold level that indicates SIBO. However, if you have a fast transit time (loose stools more than twice daily) this test may show positive when in fact it isn't (a false positive) so you do need to be mindful of this.

Treatment

There are some antibiotics such as ciprofloxacin, norfloxacin, cotrimoxazole, and rifaximin that can be used to treat SIBO. However, you will need to address the dysbiosis afterward—otherwise you could find yourself in the same mess further down the line.

CHAPTER 8

LEAKY GUT

We have been dealing mostly with physical structures that you can see with the naked eye; now, as with the liver, we have to zoom right in and take a microscopic view, looking at the cells and molecules of the small intestine. This is where the major task of absorbing all the nutrition from your food takes place, and to understand that we need to see it at a molecular level.

STRUCTURE AND FUNCTION
OF THE SMALL INTESTINE—PART TWO

When I (DD) was fourteen I took my bike apart, including the rear hub. Who knew there were all those ball bearings in it? Of course I couldn't get them all back in, and the bike was never the same. There is a similar problem when a surgeon opens up your abdomen; it's difficult to get all that intestine back inside, particularly if it's at all swollen.

Most of this is small intestine—small as in narrow, that is. As described in the last chapter, it is less than an inch (about 2.5 centimeters) or so across, although it's long, averaging over 20 feet (6 meters) in an adult. It's also big in surface area. Nature achieves that with the villi, projections like fingers that protrude into the inside of the intestine.

Villi

The reason you need all that surface area is because there are so many nutrients to be absorbed from your food. Even a fairly primitive animal like an earthworm, which is basically an intestine surrounded by a muscle, has folds and wrinkles in its intestine to increase the surface area, but our super-folded structure boosts it much more.

Zoom in closer and you can see that each of these fingerlike villi has a capillary artery bringing blood down its length to the tip, and both a vein and a lymphatic duct carrying the nutrients and other molecules away. The veins lead eventually to the portal vein, which carries everything in it to the liver for processing, storing, excreting, or building into other molecules.

GALT (Gut-Associated Lymphoid Tissue)

The lymphatic ducts, on the other hand, lead first to the gut-associated lymphoid tissue (GALT), which is the digestive system's immune system. It is made up of lymph nodes (called Peyer's patches in this part of the body) and more diffuse lymph tissues, starting with the tonsils at the back of the mouth. In fact, GALT is the single biggest set of immune tissues in the body, and for good reason; it has to tell the difference between three categories of materials it encounters:

- Food: to be absorbed and used. During the first few weeks of life, while a baby is protected by antibodies that it gets from its mother before birth and in breast milk, the GALT builds a database of nutrient molecules that will be allowed in.

- Self: to be left alone to get on with its job. You would think that this just means you, but to scientists these days it also means the microorganisms living in, on, and with you—the "friendly" bacteria. We are constantly exchanging nutrients and information with these bugs, and also using them to send information. The way you smell to others, for instance, is mostly determined by the organisms in your gut and on your skin.

- Non-self: materials that are potentially undesirable and need managing or even disposal. This includes "unfriendly" bacteria and viruses, but also a range of molecules that are in food but with which we cannot do anything useful. Dr. Leo Galland talks about a "toxic/antigenic load from which the body needs to be protected."[1]

Processing all of this food and information keeps the GALT very busy. It also means that we need an efficient screening and protection system, or else the GALT can get overloaded.

Mucus

The linings of everything in the body, from the lips to the anus, and from the nose to the bottom of the lungs, plus our urinary and reproductive parts, are all known as mucous membranes. They are called mucous (an adjective) because they are covered in mucus (a noun). This is the shiny, sometimes slimy stuff that covers and protects them, and you will only be aware of it when it comes pouring out of your nose when you have a cold.

Mucus is also a large part of what comes pouring out of somewhere else when you have diarrhea. In both cases it's the body's mechanism for ejecting something harmful. This means that (in most cases, anyway) the diarrhea or the runny nose is NOT the problem; it's the body's way of solving the problem. So suppressing it is not a smart idea—in an acute problem, that is. If the diarrhea becomes chronic you may have no choice. You may need to replace fluid and electrolytes that you have lost, but your body won't decide "better out than in" without a reason.

Healthy adults produce about a liter (a quart) of mucus every day. It is mostly made up of sugars, but not the sort that you get in a soft drink. Primitive cells started using these molecules, called glycans, so far back in evolution that they predate what we now think of as the immune system. There's a whole science now called glycobiology, or glycomics. These glycans are often mixed and combined with proteins, amino acids, and lipids, and they have two important properties: they form long chains, or polymers; and they attract huge amounts of water. That is just about all you need to make mucus.

The other half of the story is that organisms developed molecules called lectins to interact with the glycans to break them open or to bind to them. Just as antibodies are molecules that identify and react to proteins, lectins identify and react to carbohydrates, to glycans. Lectins guide where cells go in the growing embryo; the whole mechanism of ABO blood groups is based on lectins; the C-reactive protein (CRP) that your doctor uses to test for inflammation is a lectin. Essential for life and health, in other words, but sometimes they can work against us. For instance, lectins are the reason we have to cook certain beans more thoroughly or they can make us ill.

There are some parts of the digestive tract that obviously need protecting by mucus. The esophagus needs protection from scratching by sharp pieces of food, and the stomach needs protecting from its own acid. Things are less dramatic in the small intestine, but you still need protection: from infections, from drugs like aspirin, even sometimes from food (the wheat plus flu story, further down, is a good example of this). In the large bowel mucus does form a pretty much impenetrable barrier, but in the small intestines it's actually porous because your food needs to get through it in order to be absorbed. Without that protection you could easily set off inflammation of the cells, and this can easily become a self-perpetuating cycle. As we write this book a paper has just been published, reporting that when components in the mucus layer in the small intestine come in contact with the underlying cells they prevent that inflammation from happening by blocking the genes that would set it off.[2] Score another point to nature.

Cells and Junctions

The cells lining the intestine turn over faster than any other cells in the body, which gives another layer of protection from chemical damage. It is said that the intestine is in a constant state of controlled inflammation, and the primary purpose of all inflammation is healing and repair. The cells, and even more the junctions between them, need to be kept in a good state of repair or the toxic/antigenic load may get into the body. That is the condition known as leaky gut syndrome.

The junctions between cells are complex and wonderful. Do a search online for an image of "desmosomes" and you will see what we mean; nature invented Velcro way before we did. As well as the tight junctions that keep molecules above a certain size from squeezing into the body between the cells, the communicating or gap junctions create tiny channels connecting the insides of adjacent cells, through which messenger molecules can travel. This cell-to-cell communication enables cells to operate as a community, preventing individual cells from going rogue and becoming cancerous, for instance. It is also important for communication between nerve cells both in the brain and in the heart.

You can see that there are multiple defense layers between the materials coming from outside the body to inside the intestine and the inside of the body. Starting from within the intestine (closest to the "outside" materials it holds), we have:

- The mucus layer, coating and protecting the intestine

- Epithelial cells, deciding which molecules to let in

- GALT, the immune system maintaining surveillance on the incoming molecules

- The liver, filtering out the undesirables and using the good stuff

Leaky Gut

Anything that damages these layers, even just one of them, can set up a chain reaction that damages them all and breaches the intestinal barrier. Often this becomes a self-perpetuating vicious cycle that continues until an effective treatment is applied.

We could not talk about leaky gut without acknowledging the work of Dr. Leo Galland in New York; he is the go-to guy on this subject. It is clear from the research that he has brought together that if you have a leaky gut, you almost certainly have a vicious cycle going on.[3] He describes four different vicious cycles (they can coexist of course). These are liver stress, malnutrition, allergy and intolerance, and dysbiosis or SIBO (small intestinal bacterial overgrowth).

Liver Stress

It may not take much to make your gut leaky to begin with: a bout of flu or overdoing the alcohol in a serious way, for instance. When this happens, a lot of food components get absorbed that should not have been absorbed. They are taken straight to the liver, which attempts to inactivate them and excrete them in the bile. But the enzymes that perform this function can get overloaded, in which case the bile will contain both inactivated and still-active toxins. Within an hour or so of you eating it, the mix of food toxins will have been absorbed and then excreted again, damaging the intestine for a second time.

Malnutrition

It is damage to the junctions between cells that makes the intestine leaky. Whatever causes such damage is also likely to damage the rest of the cell structure and function, and, as a result, limit the active absorption of nutrients. A lot of nutrients are needed to make new cells, and the cells with the fastest turnover in the body are those lining the intestine, so a lack of nutrients will affect them first. The cells are unable to heal properly so the leak does not get fixed, and nutrient absorption does not improve.

Allergy and Intolerance

If you react to a food at its portal of entry, the intestine, this will inflame it and very likely increase its permeability. That allows food molecules to get through to trigger the immune system and set off allergic symptoms elsewhere in the body, which could range from migraines to asthma to arthritis. This keeps the immune system "irritated" and, in turn, increases its impact on the intestine.

Dysbiosis or SIBO (Small Intestinal Bacterial Overgrowth)

The list of agents that can set off this process is long, but they all fall into two categories, organisms and molecules.

Organisms. This category covers a broad range of organisms, some described in previous chapters:

- Viruses: norovirus, rotavirus, you name it, but definitely including influenza

- Bacteria: particularly acute infections such as gastroenteritis

- Yeasts: candida and other organisms can dig into the bowel lining, but their main damage is done by inhibiting the "friendly" bacteria

- Parasites: *Giardia, Blastocystis,* and others that you may not know you are carrying in your intestine

We don't want to get into the role of infections too much, but it should be pretty clear that a norovirus that gives you vomiting and diarrhea isn't kind to your gut wall.

Molecules. Molecules also can play a role in damage to your gut, including:

- Alcohol: if you ever drank with a rugby team you know what we mean. It's not rocket science.

- Non-steroidal anti-inflammatory drugs (NSAIDs): because they inhibit inflammation and repair, especially at the point of entry into the body. It only takes a single dose of aspirin or acetaminophen to increase the gut permeability short term.

- Heavy metals: it turns out that nickel, especially, can be really bad for the gut (see below)

- Wheat and gluten: these can be harmful in so many ways (see next section)

Zac was twenty-one, and a bright student, bright enough to win a scholarship to go and study in Guadalajara for a year. He already had some fairly minor health issues; in fact, he had diagnosed his own lactose intolerance as the cause of his irregular bowel function and general lack of energy and zing. Cutting out all dairy products had fixed it.

Only two weeks into the Mexico stay he developed acute diarrhea and vomiting. An antibiotic took the edge off this but left him with chronic loose bowels, bloating, and discomfort. Three more courses of antibiotic didn't fix it, and aside from the abdominal symptoms he was often weak, dizzy, and prone to dehydration. If anybody did a biochemistry panel on him while he was there I (DD) never heard about it—a pity, as it would probably have shown that his electrolytes were a mess. Diarrhea or vomiting does that to you.

So he got back home, to a diet he was more accustomed to, and things settled down a bit more, but not much. He was pretty independent, so he started cutting out various foods to see if it helped. Sometimes it did, but his response to things kept changing, and the list of foods to avoid kept growing. By the time he came to see me he was on two antidiarrheal medications most days.

We ran a panel of tests and they showed several interesting, connected things: As suspected, his gut permeability (leakiness) was very high, almost off the scale. There was a lot of fat in his stools, even though he was already on a low-fat diet (because it helped his symptoms), so leakiness was not the only consequence of his illness and treatment—he also had fat malabsorption. His blood vitamin D was seriously low; since it's a fat-soluble vitamin, not absorbing fats meant he didn't absorb vitamin D either. Which meant it wouldn't help repair his gut at all. He had none of the healthy (perhaps essential) *Lactobacillus* organisms in his large bowel, as a result of all the antibiotics.

A couple of minor rises in liver enzymes suggested that the liver was starting to get clogged up, so the cumulative effects were starting.

> All of this meant treatment was pretty easy. We kept him off the foods that disagreed with him (for now) and started him on Vitamin D, glutamine, zinc, phosphatidylcholine, and probiotics.
>
> At the time of writing he is still under treatment and doing well, feeling better week by week.

- Food allergens: reactions to foods can both be caused by and cause leaky gut—a classic self-sustaining cycle.

- Genetically-modified foods: many contain toxins, such as *Bacillus thuringiensis* (Bt) toxin that are intended to harm the gut of pest insects, and almost certainly harm ours just the same.

WHEAT-ASSOCIATED DISEASES

As early humans were migrating out of East Africa around 10,000 years ago, they all had to pass through the so-called fertile triangle in the Middle East. It was there that they picked up the trick of harvesting and eating the seeds of a grass that we now call wheat. This was the birth of agriculture. It's strange that it was only 70 years ago that we figured out that wheat might be bad for us sometimes. We had known about celiac syndrome, also called sprue, for some time, but we didn't know what caused it. (The word celiac just means abdominal, and sprue is an old Dutch word for a chronic gut problem.) Then, in the 1940s, a Dutch pediatrician named Dicke figured out that giving wheat to children with celiac made their symptoms worse.

In the 1960s it all started to come together; first a researcher found evidence of antibodies to gluten in people with celiac disease. A skin disease, dermatitis herpetiformis, and then some neurological diseases were also linked to wheat. Since then we have come to realize that there are a range of different reactions to wheat, and we have worked out the mechanism pretty well. This just leaves one question to answer: if wheat can make us ill in all these different ways, is the reaction to it the problem or the body's attempt at a solution?

Gluten and Celiac Disease

Gluten just means glue in Latin. It is a storage protein that the wheat seed plans to use when it starts growing, but when you make bread from wheat flour it is the gluten that makes it softer, lighter, and better to eat. Naturally, humans have always tried to increase the gluten content of the flour they use, but it's only in the last fifty or so years that we've got really good at this. That's around the same time that we have seen something of an explosion in the occurrence of reactions to it.

Celiac disease is an autoimmune disease triggered by exposure to gluten.[4] Specifically (and slightly more simply than in real life) there is a fragment of gluten known as the 33-mer (because it is 33 amino acids long) that is surprisingly resistant to all the digestive enzymes and thus stands a chance of getting through to the immune system, the GALT. There it can set off an immune reaction, but this is only really a problem in people who have specific gene types. If you have one of these gene types, known as HLA DQ2 and HLA DQ8, then you make cell surface receptors (proteins on the outer surface of your cells) that are similar enough to the 33-mer that once your immune system reacts to 33-mer it may react to your own receptors. That is when it gets harmful. This immune reaction particularly attacks the cells lining the small intestine, and an increase in gut permeability—leaky gut—is one of the earliest changes that result.

The "classic" symptoms of celiac disease are chronic diarrhea, abdominal discomfort, weight loss, and fatigue. Note that this illness has had an "upgrade" from syndrome to disease because syndrome means "we know these symptoms happen together but we don't know why," and now we do know what causes them. That list of symptoms always included some non-gut ones such as anemia and osteoporosis, and the big one, neurological disorders.

You need to have either a HLA DQ2 or a HLA DQ8 gene—as do about 25 percent of Caucasians—to develop true celiac, but if you do have the gene *and* you do eat wheat there is only a 30 percent chance that you will develop celiac at some time in your life. For this reason a positive gene test proves nothing, whereas a negative gene test proves that you cannot have celiac—although there are plenty of other wheat-triggered diseases you could have. Antibody tests can confirm if you have celiac, and about 1 percent of the population tests positive at any time.

Doctors used to think (maybe some still do) that it was an "on" or "off" situation: either you had full-scale celiac disease or you were probably making it up. But now we know two things for sure: firstly, that for every person who is seriously ill with celiac disease there are a number with a much less severe version; and secondly, that there are a number of other ways in which wheat can make you ill—which we will cover now.

Gluten Ataxia

Gluten and celiac were first linked to nerve diseases back in the 1960s, but it was not until 1996 that the connection was properly worked out, mostly by a small team of neurologists in the English city of Sheffield.[5] It came to be called gluten ataxia because this was the first group of patients they identified, but they have now described several different neurological disorders that are linked to a reaction to gluten. About 40 percent of patients have ataxia, an unsteadiness and lack of coordination, sometimes with involuntary movements, due to changes in the cerebellum, the part of the brain that controls movement. Another 40 percent have neuropathy: alterations in sensation, problems controlling movement, or both, caused by changes in nerves, not in the brain. The remaining 20 percent is made up of small numbers of patients with migraine, epilepsy, myopathy (muscular weakness), and stiff person syndrome (a thankfully rare disease that waxes and wanes but inexorably progresses, with stiffness and spasms of all the muscles).

When these neurologists compared their statistics with the gastroenterology department, they figured out that, for every four people diagnosed with a gluten problem in the gut, there was one with a gluten problem in the nervous system. What's more, if you have an unexplained (meaning undiagnosed) neurological disease, there is about a 50 percent chance that it is due to a gluten problem.

Wheat Allergy/Intolerance

There are three times as many people who don't have those HLA genes as those who do, and there are many more proteins in wheat than just gluten. So it would be logical for there to be more people with wheat allergy or wheat intolerance than celiac, and so there are. You just can't rely on the blood tests or even skin tests, though, so the published papers on this are completely unreliable. We believe a best guess would be that about 10 percent of the population has a reaction to wheat. That's ten times more than those who have celiac.

Symptoms of a wheat allergy may be digestive, such as abdominal bloating and discomfort, erratic bowel function, and/or more general symptoms such as tiredness, fuzzy headedness, problems with concentration and memory, general sluggishness, and disturbance of sleep.

There is also a diagnosis with one of the longest names we know: wheat-dependent exercise-induced anaphylaxis (WDEIA). The name does describe it clearly, though. It commonly happens to runners who, partway through a run or race, and at no other time, develop an allergic reaction. This is often urticaria (hives) but sometimes even can be a life-threatening anaphylactic reaction.

Wheat Germ Agglutinin

There is one more problem that wheat can cause in pretty much anyone, and it also requires two factors to come together. Wheat germ agglutinin (WGA) is a lectin, and wheat germ has a lot of it on its surface because it helps to protect the plant's cells against bacteria and fungi. This is because the lectin is specific to a glycan called N-acetyl glucosamine (NAG), and there is a lot of NAG in the cell walls of fungi and bacteria. There is also a lot of NAG on the surfaces of the epithelial cells lining the gut, so WGA is capable of attacking and harming these cells but normally can't get to them because of the mucus layer.

WGA, like the gluten 33-mer, is not broken down by cooking or by our digestive enzymes, so the mucus is our only protection against it. And there is ten times as much of it in whole-grain flour as there is in white flour, making it one more reason why whole grain may not always be better for us.

Now, the influenza virus also has a lot of lectins on its surface, and two of these lectins are important for this story. Their names are unhelpful, so we will just call them by their initials, H and N. H binds to one of the glycans in the mucus of the gut and holds the virus stable while N attacks and splits the glycans.

When this happens it breaks open the mucus layer and lets the food lectins such as WGA reach the epithelial cells. The WGA sets off defensive inflammation, and any inflamed tissue is swollen and more porous, so already you have a leaky gut. But there is more: young, newly made cells have a lot of glycans on the surface, which they lose gradually as they age. Inflammation keeps the cell population young, however. This gives the lectins more to work on and so perpetuates the cycle of inflammation.

There is a sequel to this story too; once the gut has been made leaky the WGA can get through into the bloodstream. The NAG to which it is specific is found in large quantities in cartilage, and, when the WGA binds to it there, it can cause inflammation of the joints, arthritis. That is why people take glucosamine for arthritis—to lure the WGA away from joints by giving it something else to which to bind. It works sometimes, but you do have to take a lot of glucosamine every day. Of course, cutting out wheat is likely to help too. WGA can also attack the kidneys, binding to and damaging its tissues. A 2007 study found that the people who ate the most bread had twice the risk of developing kidney cell cancer.

Remember cholecystokinin, the hormone produced when food hits the duodenum, activating the pancreas and gallbladder to produce their digestive juices? It also makes you feel full and suppresses the appetite. But WGA can bind to and block this receptor, preventing cholecystokinin from working. This means your appetite does not switch off as it should, nor do you produce digestive enzymes and bile when you should, so you don't absorb the nutrients in your food properly. This malabsorption affects oils (lipids) more than carbohydrate or protein and can lead to deficiencies of both oils and fat-soluble vitamins. And if you're still hungry, but fatty foods don't seem to agree with you, and anyway you've been told they give you heart disease (they don't), what are you going to snack on?

Nickel

This metal is well-known as a cause of contact dermatitis, typically reactions to metal in clothing, but researchers only recently (2009) described systemic nickel allergy syndrome (SNAS).[6] This gives you the skin rash plus headaches and gut problems.

You can find nickel in any non-precious metal—that's any metal apart from high-purity gold or silver—so you can be exposed by rings and jewelry, watchstraps, jeans buttons, bra clips, and so on. But the best way to get a sharp dose of nickel is with a non-precious piercing, whether for an earring or a belly-button stud. Of course it is in some dental materials, and in metal implants such as artificial hips and knees, and allergy to these is a recognized problem. It's even in some replacement heart valves.

Nickel is a component of stainless steel and can leak out of stainless pots and pans during cooking. It can get into drinking water although this is uncommon unless you are off the grid and have your own source of water. There is disagreement about which foods contain a high nickel content, which probably reflects local variations. The only good agreement seems to be about cocoa/chocolate and cashew nuts (which seems a real shame). You will get nickel from smoking too, along with cadmium, but in fact there is significantly more nickel in electronic cigarettes than in the real ones—tiny nanoparticles of nickel and tin.[7]

Why does this matter? Nickel seriously damages the gut wall. According to animal studies it simultaneously causes oxidative damage and kills the enzymes that should repair that damage. This sets off a cycle of inflammation; you could think of it as being the internal equivalent of the contact dermatitis. This is known as systemic nickel allergy syndrome, and it has three clusters of symptoms, including contact dermatitis, headaches, and gastrointestinal symptoms such as bloating, flaulence, generally erratic bowel habits, and abdominal discomfort.

But there is an additional effect as well: when they tested people with SNAS for lactose intolerance, 75 percent of them were positive,[8] compared to only 7 percent of the controls (people without a nickel problem). Lactose intolerance isn't an allergy; it is caused by an enzyme deficiency. Although lactase is a digestive enzyme, it doesn't come from the pancreas, it is produced by the cells lining the small intestine. Clearly, the nickel is hurting these cells so much that they can't produce either lactase or the antioxidant enzymes.

Nickel has been with us for a long, long time and we have been aware that it causes contact dermatitis for a long time. But why have we only just figured out SNAS? Probably because of the rise of both piercings and prostheses—multiple piercings, that is, rather than just a tasteful pair of earrings, and more and more joints, valves, and other prostheses in more and more people. Also, the rate of nickel allergy is 17 percent in women and only 3 percent in men; doctors assume this is because women have more contact with jewelry, but we don't really know.

Treatment

Your doctor may well prescribe steroid creams for a nickel rash, and this is reasonable at least in the short term. Keep on doing it for too long, though, and the adverse effects will outweigh the benefits. It won't do anything if you have a nickel problem in your gut however. In this case there are two things you should do before moving on to the general treatment of leaky gut: Avoid nickel from any source, to reduce your ongoing exposure, and take lots of zinc by mouth, which will gradually displace nickel from the body in general and the gut in particular.

CHAPTER 9

THE LARGE INTESTINE AND ITS GOINGS ON OR OUT

We are still in that long tube of the digestive system, only now we are inside the last six feet of the gastrointestinal (GI) tract, lovingly referred to as either the colon, large bowel, or large intestine. This last bit, in two dimensions, looks like a bike tire. It's a good thing that it doesn't puncture like my tires, or we would be in real difficulty.

STRUCTURE AND FUNCTION OF THE LARGE INTESTINE

The colon begins at the ileocecal valve; that's the valve between the small (ileum) and large intestine. If you have inflammatory bowel disease you can often feel a bit of discomfort if you palpate this. Go on, give it a try; you will find yours on the right hand side of your abdomen halfway between the top of your hipbone and your navel. It gets its name from where it lies: between the ileum and the cecum (the first part of the large intestine). A little bit lower down at the end of the cecum is the appendix. That's a little wormlike structure that seems to have lost its function through the process of evolution. Some scientists believe its purpose is to house beneficial bacteria to release in times of infection.[1] Fat chance of that on a Westernized diet. Charles Darwin proposed that the appendix was used to digest leaves as primates. Herbivores such as horses and koala bears still have a very long cecum, suggesting Darwin's theory might be correct. Moving right along, we have the ascending colon going up the right-hand side of the abdomen. A 90 degree turn takes us along the abdomen just under the navel inside the transverse colon, and then the colon descends, after another 90 degree turn, down the left-hand side of the abdomen. The sigmoid colon, a curly portion like a letter *c*, finishes in the rectum. The anal sphincter ensures that all the waste stays in place until we can run to the toilet. The areas of the large intestine that come under a lot of stress include the rectum and the sigmoid colon because waste products tend to spend a while here before they are excreted. Some of us don't really receive the appropriate signals to give us the "urge" and others of us ignore the urge until it's convenient. I (AP) really don't recommend this as a regular thing to do.

Now that you can see your way along this last part of the inner tube; what actually makes it work? To begin with, it has four layers to its overall structure. The outside layer, which is in contact with other organs, is a serous layer. All organs are covered with this serous layer to allow friction-free movement in close proximity to other organs. (We talked about this earlier in the book.) The Chinese will tell you it helps to get Qi energy between the organs. The rectum is exempt from the serous layer because it doesn't move much. Just below the serous layer is the lamina propria, or muscle layer. If you remember, peristalsis (a wavelike motion) is extremely important in the bowel to ensure that the stool moves forward and is expelled. The layer below the muscle is the submucosa, which contains connective tissue, glands, lymphatic vessels, and nerves. Have you noticed how the bowel misbehaves when you are nervous? It's all to do with our old friend the vagus nerve doing its wandering again. The innermost layer is the gastric mucosa, so again a mucus-secreting layer protects from erosion and bacterial invasion.

The main function of the bowel is to absorb fluids and some nutrients from the stool to ensure that the stool is fairly solid so it can be propelled out of the body. Not too solid, mind, or it won't exit very fast and you will feel somewhat lousy. In the small intestine the stool is liquid; if it remains so you will suffer from continual urgency—not good if you want to get on with life. The bacteria in the colon (bifidobacterium) break down some digestive material even further.

Mucus is also produced at the end of the digestive tract to ensure a smooth passage for your stool. If this doesn't happen for any reason, you may have to take mucilaginous foods to help the process. (More on these later, in the treatment and recipes sections.)

Elimination or defecation is the name given to the expulsion of the digestive residues we call feces or stools. This is a reflex action that occurs when the rectum becomes full, stimulating receptors in the rectal mucosa. The rectum is normally empty until a major wave of peristalsis moves fecal matter out of the colon into the rectum. It's like watching the waves come onto the beach, washing up all the pebbles and empty shells. In simplistic terms the minerals calcium and magnesium work like an orchestra, balancing contraction and relaxation of the muscles, creating the peristalsis. It is worth noting that some of this reflex is under voluntary control. If you inhibit defecation you are asking for trouble because the receptors soon become depressed, and the urge will go away until hours later, at the next point when the waves wash up the seabed debris again. Constipation occurs when the stool moves along the colon way too slowly. Extra water is then absorbed from the colon creating a hard, dry stool, and again you feel lousy. The reason you feel lousy is because, if the toxins from the compost heap of feces are not expelled, they get reabsorbed and recycled. Diarrhea may also occur when food waste travels too fast through the small intestine, or when foods you cannot digest well cause irritation and inflammation of the bowel wall. The acid chyme (remember from the stomach?) moves through the intestine too quickly, reducing the amount of absorption of fluids and electrolytes. Bacterial overgrowth (SIBO) toxins may damage the water reabsorption mechanisms, further exacerbating diarrhea. This can be fatal for infants as they have minimal fluid and electrolyte reserves. It's not that great for you either, if you miss your bus because you can't get off the toilet in the morning.

Inflammatory Bowel Disease

Remember as a kid you ran around playing tag? If you were unlucky or particularly clumsy you might trip on the pavement and fall, taking the skin off your knees and the heels of your palms. Do you also remember how inflamed it became as your immune system sent loads of white blood cells to the area to fight off any invading bacteria? The area became swollen and sore, maybe even weepy. Well, this is what happens in inflammatory bowel disease, only it's on the inside. You cannot see it, but, by golly, can you feel it. For some of you the burning sensation will be too much to bear. For others the symptoms may be so subtle as to prevent you from wearing tight clothes.

When I remember all the kids with autism spectrum disorders that I have worked with, not one of them liked to wear jeans or tightly fitting clothes. Every one of them liked soft fabrics, preferably two sizes bigger than required. Others either stripped their clothes off or turned them inside out. Some of this was the result of sensory overload, but some was the result of bowel inflammation that they couldn't verbalize because they had no baseline of good health. It's amazing how a few dietary changes of the type we will show you made all the difference. Dr. Andrew Wakefield has uncovered some groundbreaking research in the area, in case you are looking for further reading. If you have inflammatory bowel disease and a kid with autism, then you should be reading further.

Your imagination should be running riot now, with a clear visual of the inside of an excoriated (abraded) bowel. So what does it mean exactly? Well, inflammatory bowel disease (IBD) is a general term for a number of chronic conditions of the intestines associated with inflammation that can exacerbate or go into remission seemingly without reason or causation. The two most common types are Crohn's disease and ulcerative colitis.

In Crohn's disease it's the final part of the small intestine that is usually affected, but it can affect any part of the whole digestive tract from the mouth to the anus. It can also find its way onto the outside walls of the bowel in the mesentery (the outside covering of the intestines) or the lymph nodes in the area. In ulcerative colitis the inside walls of the colon or large intestine are the points of origin. IBD seems to occur between the ages of fifteen and thirty-five years with women being slightly more affected than men. It most certainly has been on the increase since the end of World War II, so Westernization has a part to play in its inception. This has been supported in Asian studies, as Asian populations are now having an explosion of IBD since they have Westernized. Although the cause of IBD is still seen as idiopathic (with no known cause), there does seem to be a genetic predisposition followed by an exaggerated immune response to some kind of environmental trigger. That might be an infection such as *Mycobacterium paratuberculosis* from unpasteurized cow's milk. Most of the milk in the United States and the United Kingdom is pasteurized now, so there must be another source if this is one of those bugs we need concern ourselves about. Other infections, such as viral insults like rotavirus, Epstein-Barr, and cytomegalovirus, and not forgetting pseudomonas-like organisms such as Chlamydia and *Yersinia enterocolitica,* may be responsible.

There is a bit of a difference between these two conditions that you need to know about. Ulcerative colitis manifests with abdominal pain, diarrhea, and hematochezia (fresh bleeding from the anus). It can be rectum and sigmoid (left-sided), extensive (up the sigmoid and across the transverse colon), or pancolitis (the entire colon). Some poor souls have to have their colon removed to gain any quality of life. In Crohn's disease the inflammation is characteristically transmural (migrating through the entire wall of the bowel) and resembles aphthous ulcers (just like the ones in the mouth) on a bed of cobblestones. Abdominal pain that seriously limits nutrient intake is a key feature. Diarrhea as a result of severe mucosal injury is prominent, alongside malabsorption of fats, fat-soluble vitamins, loss of fluids and electrolytes, and minerals. The weight loss can be catastrophic. Even though we have really good methods of detection it is still often difficult to differentiate between the two conditions. Interestingly, when the pre-illness diets of patients with Crohn's disease and ulcerative colitis were analyzed, Crohn's patients were found to have a history of refined-carbohydrate-heavy diets compared to controls, while those with ulcerative colitis didn't. It may well be that food allergy or intolerance is the key factor in ulcerative colitis. Gluten would be the likely responsible food here. (We have discussed celiac disease and gluten sensitivity in the previous chapter, so feel free to reread this information.)

Complications of IBD

Malnutrition and unhealthy weight loss occurs in about 65 percent of patients with IBD. Eating less is the most common cause, since the symptoms of inflammation put you off eating. You seem to react to anything and everything. Essential minerals and electrolytes lost through constant diarrhea can leave you weak, as can the inability to digest and absorb fats. This is especially so for anyone who has had a resection of the small intestine because less surface area means less absorption and less enzyme and bile salt activity. The end result is potential fat-soluble vitamin deficiency (vitamins A, D, E, and K) and associated health issues. Even with increased protein intake the turnover of intestinal cells ups the demand for protein. This cannot be met by the impaired cells, so protein malnutrition may be obvious.

Iron depletion and anemia are also commonplace due to possible low stomach acid or chronic loss of blood. Common drugs such as corticosteroids add to the burden by stimulating protein breakdown, depressing protein synthesis, decreasing absorption of calcium and phosphorus, and increasing urinary excretion of vitamin C, calcium, and potassium. Zinc, B_{12}, and folate deficiencies are also worth noting. No wonder these patients sometimes resemble concentration camp victims. This really is not a good place to be, but hopefully with our help you can turn your condition around.

How Come There Is So Much Inflammation?

Mononuclear and polymorphonuclear leukocytes (specialized white blood cells) head to the excoriated areas of the intestines or other sites of injury to mount an attack on the perceived invader. Remember that fall on the pavement we talked about earlier? Inflammation is the body's normal response to injury so in this case it is doing its job. The problem is that these cells (we call them pro-inflammatory mediators) recruit other cells to assist them. Activation of a protein complex called NF kappa B (NFkB), which normally regulates the immune response, gets a little overexpressive. There is an army of other cells involved in fighting inflammation too: interferon-γ, interleukins, eicosanoids, thromboxanes, and leukotrines class 4. NFkB is an aid to stimulate the release of these, in addition to stimulating molecules that protect the host from inflammation. It isn't important for you to memorize all these fancy names (but you could do it to win the pub quiz, or bore your friends). Genetics and dietary intake can influence NFkB activation, in particular butyrate, polyphenols, and essential fatty acids.

Maybe I need to say a little more about fatty acids because we are all fixated on omega-3 as being the "good guy" that's quells inflammation. However, in trials on people with psoriasis, too much omega-3 has been shown to depress the immune system. Drs. Patricia and Ed Kane have uncovered some amazing work on the appropriate balance of essential fats for the body and their belief is that a 4:1 ratio of omega-6 (linoleic acid) to omega-3 (alpha linolenic acid) is optimal.[2] This is our approach in clinical practice and it seems to work well.

You have to scrap all the hype on omega-6 because the media would have us believe that we get enough omega-6 from our food. The problem is that animal fats and trans fats are all included in that calculation. We don't see many patients in our clinic who use cold-pressed good quality omega-6 oils. For the most part, it's found in their frying pan. Its benefits are lost when heated, as the oils become damaged. (I would love to spend the next week showing you this, but it would take us off track and I may get too evangelistic.) I have another little pearl to tell you about in the form of phosphatidyl-choline, but I will get to that later.

Let me get back to butyrate, because this is another amazing fat. In fact, it's a short chain fatty acid (SCFA). Some studies have shown it to be important in reducing cytokines,[3] thereby reducing inflammation, while others have shown it to increase gene expression.[4] Butyrate feeds the colonic mucosa. Normally it would be produced by the commensal or beneficial bacteria in the colon, but these are in short supply in IBD, which further exacerbates the disease. This offers a clear benefit for their use in IBD cases.

Potential Implications of Malabsorption in IBD

Malabsorption and malnutrition of the type seen in IBD can have catastrophic effects. In children it can manifest as stunted growth and weight loss with loss of muscle mass. These patients may endure a poor quality of life, plagued with depression and anxiety. Remember the direct gut-brain link? Bone health may also suffer, due to calcium and vitamin D deficiency. The prevalence for osteopenia is around 50 percent, with 15 percent of patients going on to develop osteoporosis. Anemia is commonplace and can be due to iron, B_{12}, and folic acid deficiency. High levels of homocysteine are also often seen in IBD, again due to malabsorption of B_{12} and folate.[5] Annual testing for B_{12} levels via a methylmalonic acid (MMA) test should be performed yearly.

Phosphatidylcholine for Mucosal Protection

OK, so we promised you a pearl, and here it is: Remember we discussed the role of the mucous membranes in IBD? We are going to go into this a little more now. The mucous membrane in the colon serves a useful purpose as the first barrier of protection from the invasion of bacteria in the stool. We know we cannot avoid the bacteria, so the best solution is to protect the delicate intestinal cells. Interestingly, according to Stremmel, mucous is derived from phospholipids, of which phosphatidylcholine (PC) makes up 90 percent.[6] Lipids need to attach themselves to proteins for transport into the lumen, and it is arranged with proteins as carriers within the colon. Stremmel has shown that the PC content is reduced by 70 percent in cases of ulcerative colitis. In three clinical trials supplementation demonstrated improvement in levels of inflammation and even resolution of IBD. Further studies have demonstrated that PC has a protective effect against the ravages of nonsteroidal anti-inflammatory drugs (NSAIDs) such as diclofenac, ibuprofen, naproxen, celecoxib, mefenamic acid, etoricoxib, indomethacin, and aspirin in doses greater than 600 milligrams (mg) per day. We know these drugs damage the gut lining, reducing gut integrity.[7] This is an exciting development in the search for a natural therapy that may be influential in the reduction in symptomatology of ulcerative colitis. PC has been shown to be secreted in the ileum passing into the colon so the lowest concentration of PC is in the rectum. This may explain the clinical presentation of ulcerative colitis being primarily in the rectum with proliferation to other parts of the colon. According to Gibson and Muir,[8] who also studied PC in ulcerative colitis, less PC and lysophosphatidylcholine (LPC, the other major class of phospholipids) were found in the rectal mucosa of patients with ulcerative colitis compared to either controls or patients with Crohn's disease. The authors inferred that a lack of phospholipids, either through reduced production, increased breakdown, or both could be at fault in colitis. Phospholipids are absorbed by the mucus so their presence can be significantly increased by topical application. There is a school of thought that the supplements need to be enteric coated to reach the colon, however. The alternative is to consider phospholipid enemas. We call this bottoms up therapy!

Probiotics for Improvement in Barrier Function

Probiotics have been studied for more than two decades. There is very strong evidence to support their role in reducing bowel inflammation in those who are genetically predisposed to IBD. As much as we have seen promising results in mixed-strain delivery of probiotic bacteria it is difficult to find strain-specific results. That said, the results for ulcerative colitis are promising in that prevention of relapse, and treatment in mild to moderate attacks, has yielded good results. VSL#3 (bifidobacterium and lactobacillus) appears to be the probiotic of choice, and if you have ulcerative colitis the chances are that you can get this by prescription from your general practitioner.

This brings us to our next case:

A young man of thirty-two years of Nigerian descent presented with ulcerative colitis of three years duration. He had needed a blood transfusion following diagnosis and was treated with mesalazine and prednisolone. He was later switched to sulphasalazine when his joints began to swell, especially in his ankles and fingers. This kept his colitis under control, but sadly for him one of the side effects of the drug can be kidney problems, and he was unlucky in that department. Two years after his diagnosis an attack of food poisoning upset the balance for his colitis, and he was hospitalized again. He was discharged on azothioprine and prednisolone, and this was when the young man came to see us. A comprehensive biochemistry panel highlighted high cholesterol, low iron, and raised urea and creatinine levels. His glomerular filtration rate was 53, below the normal level of 60, so this was another good indication that his kidneys were struggling somewhat. We also ran a gut permeability panel; while this is not viewed as diagnostic for malabsorption it offers valuable information that might reflect impaired absorption due to atrophy or fibrosis.

This young man was treated initially with vitamin D at 10,000 mg per day (based on his skin color and residence—he was dark skinned and living in the United Kingdom, so one would expect his levels to be low.) Within a week the bleeding had ceased and bowel habits had improved. His vitamin D levels came up nicely on the next testing session. Dietary measures were high-fat, low-carb from lipid- and protein-rich foods (of the type we will discuss later). The rationale for this approach came from the work of Stremmel (discussed earlier). A probiotic called Culturelle was also added to his regimen. The young man became symptom-free very quickly. It will be important to ensure that remission continues with yearly colonoscopies as part of disease management. As we do not yet have an enteric-coated phosphatidylcholine available in the United Kingdom, a regular product was recommended and commenced.

Diverticular Disease

Diverticular disease is another inflammatory condition where the walls of the bowel become weakened and parts of the walls bulge to form sacs called diverticula. (Think back to your bike (or car) tire again; remember those bubbles on the side of the tire that burst if you didn't get to the repair shop in time?) There are a number of stages to diverticular disease. The actual condition that produces these bulges, without symptoms, is called diverticulosis. Once there is inflammation the "osis" becomes "it is," so we get diverticulitis. This is the result of toxic waste getting trapped in these diverticula, which means they become swollen and blocked. Because the symptoms are so similar this can become confused with irritable bowel syndrome (IBS). Not that IBS is a syndrome at all—it's just a term given to a collection of symptoms such as abdominal discomfort, chronic constipation, fever, nausea, vomiting, and diarrhea when no cause can be found. IBS is a disease of "civilized society" as it doesn't exist in countries where the diet is unrefined.

Most cases of diverticular disease are controlled with diet and medication, but sometimes seriously inflamed diverticula can perforate. Abscesses, pus, and bacteria on the outside of the colon wall can lead to peritonitis, which can be life threatening. Fiber deficiency seems to be the main trigger for the development of diverticula. In the past physicians have advocated that nuts and seeds should be avoided in this condition. However, according to a follow-up study by L. L. Strate and his research team, this is only necessary during the acute phase.[9] Bowel rest is encouraged during the acute phase, with soups and essential-oil-blended juices with a maximum of 10 grams (g) of fiber per day. The dietary fiber is then gradually increased, as the condition allows, by 5 g per week, up to a target intake of 25–35 g per day.

A review of the available evidence has failed to show a negative relationship between nut consumption and diverticulitis risk. Interestingly, Strate's team claims there is a protective effect from the consumption of nuts and seeds, presumably due to their essential oil content. This is great news because the power drink we used in our case above can now be used with diverticular disease cases. The nuts and seeds in the drink have been soaked and blended to provide a nutrient-dense drink or meal replacement that doubles as a transport medium for supplements. What a find!

CONCLUSION

By now some of you will have had a meander through the digestive system from top to toe savoring and digesting every word, while others may have dipped into the chapters that were particularly relevant to them. The mucous membrane is the same from one end to the other, so there will be things you can do that may help more than one area of the digestive system. You may get a surprise when you resolve one symptom area that another resolves too. There are also things that are specific to one area only.

Our plan was to make this as simple as we could so you can use this information safely and effectively. We also wanted to make this a practical book, so to that end we have the appendices. These are the "what to do" sections, offering dietary changes and recipes, and appropriate supplements where these may be deemed necessary, along brief overviews of why we have chosen this particular approach. The flowchart in Figure 9.1 below might be a useful memory aid.

However you chose to use the material in this book, we hope it makes a difference to your digestive health and well-being.

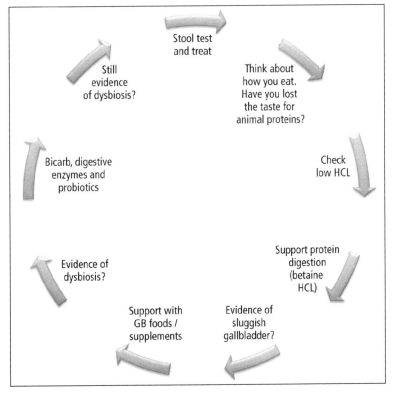

Figure 9.1 Digestive algorithm

NUTRITIONAL APPROACH

Now that we have hopefully helped you to understand the difference between normal and dysfunctional workings of your digestion, this is where you commit to changing yours. It is beyond the scope of the book to offer every recipe you are likely to need, but we have included our tried and tested "know that works" recipes to get you started.

Before we talk about dietary changes it would probably be helpful if we explained why you need to follow this diet, and what on earth the rationale is behind it all. There is no way you will follow this regimen if you can't see the point, so here goes. This is literally a high-fat, low-carb (HFLC) diet. Ouch, our ears! We can hear you screaming from here, but please just hold on a short while. We need to tell you this next bit. We have been brainwashed for such a long time regarding a low-fat diet and its value for weight loss, diabetes, cardiovascular health, metabolic syndrome, diabetes, and a host of other conditions. These are not important to you right now but the concept of HFLC is, and this is why. We can't begin to tell you how many patients we see in our clinic with varying degrees of fat deficiency due to this media hype and old research that some professionals still hold onto as if it were their bible.

It isn't just the digestive system that needs these fats; it's every cell in the body. All cells have a semipermeable membrane made from phospholipids (remember, we talked a lot about phospholipids in the IBD section of the book). It is quite clear that these phospholipids are important in encouraging mucous secretion to prevent damage to the intestinal cells from the digestive juices, drugs, and other exogenous substances it encounters. Well, in other cells the semipermeable structure enables nutrients to pass into the cells and waste to pass out. Without an adequate supply and the correct balance of fats and oils, these membranes destabilize and break down. We suffer nutrient loss and cells start to die, damaging more cells in turn as they create damage, like falling dominoes. The end result is ill health and aging. Health will decline wherever your weak spots are or your jeans (oops, sorry—genes) let you down.

As the saying goes, the genetics set the scene and the environment pulls the trigger. We are obviously dealing with digestion in this book, but we think you will find that you feel and see positive results in other areas when you follow this diet, the skin being the most likely. As we have said, it's the balance that is important, and the medium by which the nutrients are delivered. To this end the mainstay of our program is something called the power drink.

Before we give you the power drink recipes, though, let's take a look at the lovely foods you will need to include in your daily regimen and those you can forget about for now. We always find that the tricky aspects of the regimen are breakfast, bread replacements, and snacks, so we have combined these as a starter program for you. For general meal ideas the paleo diet or specific carbohydrate diet (SCD) recipes will provide you with more variety. Your diet should always be high-fat low-carb, so this can be SCD, Body Ecology, paleo, or modified Atkins, but our approach is NeuroLipid Keto (ketogenic). See more on this in the dietary changes section.

Note: Products mentioned by brand name can be ordered over the Internet if they are not available locally.

Foods to Include

- Organic, grass-fed (same as free-range) red meat and poultry

- Oily fish (but never farmed): only fish lower on the food chain, such as anchovies, sardines, herrings; also wild salmon (the higher on the food chain the more mercury accumulates in the meat; you wouldn't want to eat human meat, for instance)

- Organic free-range eggs

- Ground nuts and seeds, nut and seed butter, sprouted dried seeds: grinding and sprouting ensures easier digestion and absorption and maximum nutrient availability

- Well-cooked lentils—try glass noodles

- Organic butter, goat milk, yogurt, or kefir (recipe later)

- BodyBio Balance Oil or cold-pressed, extra-virgin hemp oil

- Organic coconut butter for frying and adding to the power drink (Nutiva, Higher Nature, Viridian, Coconoil)

- Soft organic cheeses—sheep or goat milk, feta, goat kefir

- Low-carbohydrate vegetables, such as organic chives, chard, cauliflower, cabbage, sprouts, green beans, green chilies, celery, onion, leeks, zucchini (courgette), broccoli, asparagus, sugar snap peas, bok choy, eggplant (aubergine), kale, Chinese cabbage

- Salads, daily—mixed (try adding two sprigs of rosemary, two halved garlic cloves, and the juice of half a lemon to your favorite oil: leave it for one week to infuse, then drizzle on salads and vegetables)

- Fresh herbs and spices

- Paleo or SCD bread (see recipes)

- Coconut wraps

- Organic fresh, unsweetened berries

- Raw crackers—many recipes and websites selling these are available on the Internet if you cannot find these locally; use the crackers with dips such as nut and seed butters (almond, sunflower, hazelnut, Brazil), hummus, guacamole, or avocado

Foods to Exclude

- All grains—bread, pasta, confectionery, flour, cereal, and, although technically not a grain, buckwheat (Don't worry, we have some tasty alternatives!)

- Starchy vegetables—corn, carrots, parsnips, potatoes (all types)

- High-carbohydrate and high-fructose fruits—bananas, grapes, and dried fruit such as raisins and dates

- Sugars—dextrose, sucrose, fructose, corn syrup, honey, table sugar

- Convenience foods and soft drinks

- Diet drinks with aspartame, sorbitol, mannitol, malitol

- Trans fats—vegetable margarine, processed oils

- Peanuts, peanut butter, peanut oil

- Monosodium glutamate—Chinese food, food flavorings, Marmite

- Commercial mayonnaise or salad dressing

How to Exclude Foods

Here are some ground rules. We are not recommending an allergen-elimination approach—at least, that's only a part of it. There are a number of interactions and vicious cycles that can build up in the gut, and we have a rule about them, built from our experience:

You cannot break a vicious cycle at just one point; it will always re-form. You have to break it at several points simultaneously.

You have to cut out the coffee that's irritating your gut, *and* the sugar that's fermenting there, *and* the medication that's making it leaky. And even repair the leak with good food and nutrients. It's an integrated approach: that's what gets results.

Why cut out *all* grains? Well, because it gets complicated trying to distinguish between the various sorts of reactions—to wheat protein (from wheat intolerance), other grains (intolerance again), gluten (celiac), or starch (because it's a carbohydrate)—not to mention unnecessary chemicals such as aspartame and monosodium glutamate (MSG), both of which have been linked to unpleasant and sometimes serious toxic reactions.

Remember that a wheat-free diet is not a gluten-free diet. There is a small amount of gluten in most other grains including barley, rye, oats (though this is argued about), and even spelt. To go gluten-free you need to avoid all of these in addition to wheat. Buckwheat is from a different plant family, though, and is free of gluten.

And a gluten-free diet is not a wheat-free diet. Gluten is most of the protein in wheat, about 80 percent of it. This protein is different from the other proteins, though, because it's bound to the starch, the carbohydrate food store that is the biggest part of the wheat seed. Making wheat gluten-free is easy: you just wash away the starch and the gluten goes with it (making gluten-free bread needs some new techniques though, so read on). But this leaves more of the other proteins per pound of flour, which could make a wheat intolerance reaction or a wheat germ agglutinin (see WGA in Chapter 8) even worse.

Is this diet just for a month, or is it for life? Well, you know what they say about diets for weight loss—you put it all back on when you stop the diet. That's pretty much true here too. What you really need is a new lifestyle, new habits—a deep fix, not a quick fix. Does this mean you can never have a glass of wine again? Heck no! When you have fixed your gut you will be able to relax and enjoy. But believe me, you should feel so much better for taking these steps that you won't even think about going back to how your diet was before.

THE THERAPEUTIC NUTRITIONAL INTERVENTION PROGRAM

This program is focused around a "5Rs" approach:

- Remove

- Replace

- Reinoculate

- Repair

- Rebalance

Remove. Eliminate foods that may be exacerbating the problem. Consider removing high FODMAP (Fermentable Oligo, Di, Monosaccarides, and Polyols) foods. These are families of short-chain carbohydrates that are generally poorly absorbed. They include:

- Lactose

- Fructose

- Fructo and galacto-oligosaccharides (fructans and galactans)

- Polyols (sorbitol, mannitol, xyltol, malitol)

Eliminate all of the above for two weeks, then challenge (add each one back into the diet) individually.

Replace. Provide digestive support (betaine, enzymes, bile salts, bicarbonate/Tri-Salts) ninety minutes after meals.

Reinoculate. Add probiotics, kefir (water and milk), and fermented foods such as sauerkraut.

Repair. Supplement with Perm A vite, Arthred, zinc, Immuno-gG (colostrum), and vitamin D.

Rebalance. Include digestive support/immune support/probiotics. Prebiotic foods include Jerusalem artichoke, chickory, onions, garlic, leeks, tomatoes, spinach, flaxseed, and legumes.

RECIPES

POWER DRINKS/NUTRIENT DELIVERY DRINKS

Neurolipid Cocktail (or Power Drink)
(With grateful thanks to Dr. Patricia Kane)

This drink needs to be made in two stages and you will need a good blender. The Vitamix or Thermomix are recommended, but they don't come cheap. Buy the best blender you can afford and if you buy a normal kitchen-grade blender be sure to blend your seed cream in short bursts so the motor doesn't get too hot. Aside from this, you are ready to go.

The beauty of this drink is that it is a nutrient-dense super food that feeds your cell membranes. If you only make one change today, this is the important change to make.

Stage One: Soaked Seed Cream

In honesty, you can use any combination of nuts and seeds that take your fancy from the food list when making this cream. However, we find this one to be well balanced.

1 cup golden linseed (Linusit Gold is the best brand)

$1/4$ cup sesame seeds

$1/4$ cup sunflower seeds

$1/4$ cup pumpkin seeds

$1/4$ cup chia seeds

1 teaspoon E-lyte Balanced Electrolyte Concentrate

Place all seeds into a bowl or jug, cover with water, and add 1 teaspoon (5 milliliters [ml]) of E-lyte Balanced Electrolyte Concentrate. Soak overnight.

Blend to a smooth paste and freeze in ice cube trays
(standard size of ice cubes varies between countries, 20 ml
in the US and 10–12 ml in the UK); we use 50 ml medicine
cups or gallipots from nursing supplies outlets). Store in the
freezer until required, defrost before using.

Stage Two

$1/2$ cup unsweetened milk (coconut, almond,
or goat/sheep milk kefir)

2 teaspoons (10 ml) BodyBio Balance Oil (or 1 tablespoon
hemp oil and 1 teaspoon sunflower oil; must be organic
cold-pressed and not high-oleic-acid sunflower oil).

2 organic free-range eggs

2 tablespoons egg protein powder
(this is freely available on the Internet,
but it's best to use at least free range if you can)

1 50 ml medicine cup or 4 12 ml (UK)
ice cubes of frozen seed cream (from Stage One)

2 teaspoons E-lyte Balanced Electrolyte Concentrate

1 to 2 teaspoons phosphatidylcholine

Mix the Stage One and Stage Two ingredients together when
ready to drink. This drink is superb taken as a meal replacement during the day or for breakfast. You can also use it to
add any supplements, especially for children. Add everything
you are trying to get into your body to the mix, then process
it in the blender for a good three minutes.

Variations: For a different flavor you could add stevia cocoa
powder, Bourbon vanilla, or a handful of frozen berries. Do
not add flavoring before blending; add it right at the end and
then process for just a few seconds more, otherwise the taste
will be lost.

Go-to-Green Smoothie

(With grateful thanks to the Hemsley sisters)

This is our go-to smoothie for those times we've been deprived of raw green food (excellent as after-flight care!) or when you need to balance an earlier rich meal. This drink is alkalizing, hydrating, cleansing, antioxidant-rich, and easy to digest—not to mention its minimal prep time. And the beauty is that, with a few simple tweaks, it can be transformed from a green smoothie to a raw green soup like a gazpacho. If you're just transitioning over to the idea of drinking your vegetables or if you have a sweeter tooth, then you might want to use two apples, especially if you're using kale in the smoothie as it's a little more bitter than young spinach leaves.

A strong blender is required to make this recipe smooth. If you don't have a strong blender peel the cucumber and ginger, use spinach rather than kale, and chop everything well before blending.

YIELD: 2–3 SERVINGS (APPROXIMATELY 750 ML/$1^1/_2$ PINTS)

$^1/_2$ medium cucumber
(200 grams [g]/7 ounces [oz])

1–2 medium apples (150–300 g/5–10 oz)

2 sticks of celery (80 g/3 oz)

70 g/$2^1/_2$ oz spinach or kale leaves (stalks removed)

$^1/_2$ large, ripe avocado (60 g/2 oz)

20 g ($^3/_4$ oz) ginger

5 g (.176 oz) dried dulse

3 g (.1 oz) parsley (a small handful)

$^1/_2$ large lemon/1 small lemon
(3 tablespoons of lemon juice)

1 teaspoon super green powder
(chlorella, spirulina, or similar)

$1^1/_4$ cup filtered water (325 ml)

To make a raw soup:

2 medium spring onions

1 medium to large garlic clove

1 small pinch of cayenne, to taste

1 pinch ($3/4$ teaspoon) of sea salt, to taste

Place the dried dulse in the blender to soak.

Wash the fresh produce, chop coarsely, and add to the blender.

Add the rest of the ingredients and the remaining water to the blender. Pulse a few times and then blend until smooth. Add more water to reach the desired consistency.

If you want a raw soup, include the savory ingredients. In colder weather, warm it gently on the stove.

Variations: For those with a sweeter tooth, use two apples in your smoothie, especially if you are using the more bitter kale.

Easy Vegetable Power Drink

YIELD: 1 SERVING

2 stalks celery

$1/3$ medium cucumber

2 kale leaves

1 head bok choy

1 kiwi fruit

1 portion seed cream (recipe above)

OR

$1/2$ avocado

1 tablespoon hemp oil (cold-pressed, extra-virgin)

1 teaspoon sunflower oil (organic cold-pressed, not high-oleic)

1 teaspoon coconut oil

Cut the vegetables into pieces for blending. For very sensitive stomachs it will be better to juice the celery, cucumber, kale, and bok choy separately first, and then add them to the blender with the kiwi and seed cream or seed cream substitute ingredients, and blend well. Juicing the vegetables will reduce the fiber content. For more robust digestive systems it is fine to simply blend all the ingredients together and enjoy. If you need to add more liquid, coconut water will add a bit of sweetness and valuable electrolytes.

Variations: You can choose your own combination of vegetables. Play around with the recipe to suit your taste.

Slow-Cooked Bone Broth

This is another very important food that grandma used to make. If you are of a certain age you will remember the lovely homemade chicken soup you were given when sick. Ever wonder why you felt better after eating it? We recommend that all of you make bone broth and add it to your dietary regimen daily. It has some wonderful health benefits we want to let you know about. Top tip: it contains gelatin, which protects and heals the mucous membrane of the digestive tract. It also improves hair and nail growth and quality. Eating soup during a chest infection is said to reduce the number of white blood cells; remember, they create inflammation. Bone broth also contains glucosamine, which can stimulate the growth of new collagen, repair damaged joints, and reduce pain and inflammation. Everyone has heard of glucosamine, and this version is natural and cheaper. The minerals calcium, phosphorous, and magnesium in the broth help your bones grow and repair. The amino acids proline and glycine in bone broth also help quell inflammation, and glycine calms the mind, keeping you sane.

Slow-Cooked Chicken Broth

YIELD: APPROXIMATELY 2 TO 3 PINTS

3 stalks celery

1 small red onion

1 small carrot

1 garlic clove

$2^1/_4$ pounds (1 kilogram) organic chicken thighs
and drumsticks, with skin on

Fiber residue from green juice
(Optional. This is the dry fibrous residue left over
from vegetable juicing.)

3 teaspoons (30 ml) E-lyte Balanced Electrolyte Concentrate

$^1/_2$ teaspoon apple cider vinegar
(this helps to remove the minerals from the bone).

Freshly ground black pepper to taste

Wash and chop the vegetables and place them in a slow
cooker with the chicken, fiber residue, if using, electrolyte
concentrate, and cider vinegar. Cover completely with filtered
water. Set the slow cooker to high and cook for 12 hours.

Remove the skin from the chicken and discard. The meat
should fall off the bones and can be eaten cold with salads
for lunch. At this point you can eat the broth as it is, or
remove the vegetables and blend them. Return them to the
broth and stir in well. Add the pepper to taste.

Variations: You could also try this with organic grass-fed beef
bones for a meatier flavor. If you roast the beef bones for
half an hour prior to making the recipe it makes for a richer
tasting broth.

Kefir

Fermented foods are invaluable for digestive health, and kefir is one of the oldest. It has been used in Eastern Europe since the 1880s and its health benefits come from a medley of *Lactobacillus* bacteria and other beneficial micro-organisms, including *Saccharomyces cerevisiae*. It can be made into kefir yogurt, and cheese (cow, sheep, goat, soy, nut, or coconut milk). If you use an alternative milk you will need to feed it cow's milk every so often because this is the kefir's preferred food.

Kefir can be purchased from a number of online resources. The solid "grains" of the starter culture resemble cauliflower, and to say a little goes a long way is an understatement. It grows beautifully if you care for it well. There are different forms of kefir for different uses; you can make kefir water, or a lovely coconut champagne from dry kefir and coconut water.

So how do you grow, use, and care for your new friend? After purchase it needs to be fed and then rest for a few days, so find it a warm place in the kitchen. Place it in a sterilized and cooled Mason or Kilner jar. Cover with preboiled and cooled milk. Place a clean paper towel over the jar top to keep it clean and to allow it to breathe. After 24 hours, drain the milk through a plastic sieve (kefir hates metal, so please stick to plastic and wood). Wash the kefir with filtered water and let it drain. Meanwhile, sterilize and cool the jar again. Place the kefir grains back in the jar to rest again. (I leave mine overnight.) Add more preboiled milk the next morning.

Many people don't bother with all the washing and resting, but I find my kefir is healthier for this. I didn't have much success when I continually fed it.

Gc-MAF

Gc-MAC is a protein that all healthy people, animals, and even micro-organisms make internally. Scientists have been studying it for twenty-five years, but only recently have figured out how to produce it as a good quality product. "MAF" stands for macrophage activating factor, and basically it does what it says—it stimulates the white blood cells, known as macrophages, to "attack" and eat cancer. The word macrophage literally means "big eater," and these are large cells that swallow up viruses, cancers, tissue debris, and so on.

There is an injectable form of Gc-MAF, for which you would need a doctor to assist you, but there is now a probiotic form that you can drink, use as mouthwash, rub into skin, or even take as an enema. Like kefir, it contains a number of different organisms, in this case modeled as nearly as possible to the bacteria a baby would acquire as it is being born. Gc-MAF is expensive, costing upward of $600 for a three-month supply (it is shipped to you frozen), so you would probably try the other suggestions in this book first, and keep it in mind as an option if they don't work.

You can buy Gc-MAF from http://www.bravoprobiotic.com in the United States or www.gcmaf.eu in Europe.

BREAKFAST

Anne's Paleo Porridge

Why have we chosen this combination of nuts and seeds for this recipe? Coconut has a good supply of plant-based saturated fats in addition to medium-chain triglycerides, which confer many health benefits.[1] Pumpkins seeds[2] have been shown to have an impressive effect on the bacterial balance of the gut. Sunflower seeds are a power-house of proteins, fats, carbohydrates, vitamins, and minerals.[3] In addition to the mucilaginous properties of Chia seeds, they have been shown to be beneficial in balancing lipid ratios (lowering choles-terol).[4] Rich in omega-3 and mucilaginous properties, linseed is also purported to be a super food[5] that has shown promise in lowering lipids. The mucilaginous properties of these two seeds aid peristalsis. They do this by absorbing water to make them gluelike in consistency. This helps to provide bulk to the stool while absorbing toxins from the gut for excretion. The essential oils contained in the seeds are soothing to the digestive system, helping the stool slide along nicely. Clinically we find this particular recipe invaluable when our patients have inflamed intestines. Sesame seeds have been shown to have antifungal and antibacterial qualities, especially with streptococcal infections.[6] Walnuts are rich in omega-3 and are known to have benefits for brain health[7]—they even look like a brain. What about the two spices, cinnamon and ginger? Well, some long-standing studies show cinnamon has good effects on blood-glucose balancing,[8] and that's a major part of what we are addressing with our nutritional approach. It would take another book to tell you about all the health benefits of ginger, but suffice to say it is a true digestive tonic, used to alleviate nausea, flatulence, bloating, constipation, and a whole lot more.[9] I will need to send you to the review for the whole story. In Chinese medicine, ginger is used to improve digestive fire, which, in English terms, means gastric acid secretion. As we said earlier in this book, that is the first crucial step in rebalancing the gut.

YIELD: 1 SERVING

1 tablespoon walnuts

1 tablespoon sesame seeds

1 tablespoon desiccated coconut

1 tablespoon sunflower seeds

1 tablespoon pumpkin seeds

1 tablespoon golden linseed

1 teaspoon chia seeds

1 teaspoon ground cinnamon

1 teaspoon ground ginger

1 cup milk of your choice (almond milk works well,
as does full-fat coconut milk)

Grind all of the seeds together. Add the cinnamon and ginger and mix all dry ingredients thoroughly. If using the Vitamix, simply add all the ingredients including the milk and blend on high for two minutes. It will be warm enough to eat. If not using a Vitamix add 1 cup milk to the dry ingredients and cook on the stove at medium heat until it is warmed through. Do not boil.

If the digestion is really poor you may wish to prepare this the night before and store in the refrigerator overnight. This helps reduce the phytate content in the seeds, improving mineral uptake. This recipe can also be eaten raw-soaked if preferred.

Variation: This recipe is lovely with a dollop of sheep yogurt and a small handful of berries.

STAPLE FOODS

Anne's Linseed Bread

YIELD: ONE 1 POUND LOAF

1 cup ground flaxseed

$1/2$ teaspoon bicarbonate of soda

$1/2$ teaspoon vitamin C crystals (plain ascorbic acid) or the juice of half a lemon

1 teaspoon E-lyte Balanced Electrolyte Concentrate

2 large organic free-range eggs, whisked

$1/4$ cup water

$1/4$ cup coconut oil (or olive oil, if you don't have coconut)

Mixed seeds to sprinkle on top (caraway, sunflower, poppy)

Preheat the oven to 350°F (180°C).

Combine all the dry ingredients (flaxseed, bicarbonate of soda, vitamin C) in a large bowl. Mix the wet ingredients together (E-lyte, egg, lemon juice, water, coconut oil) in a smaller bowl. Add the wet ingredients to the dry ones, stirring well. Allow to stand for 2 to 3 minutes to allow the batter to thicken (it still should be very wet).

Line a one-pound loaf tin with parchment paper. Pour in

the batter and sprinkle the top with seeds. Bake for 20 minutes or until a knife inserted comes out clean. Remove from the oven and cool on a wire rack.

This freezes well and can be toasted.

POWER BARS

(with grateful thanks to Dr. Patricia Kane)

Butterscotch Pecan Power Bars

YIELD: 12 BARS

5 ounces organic coconut butter (Nutiva, Omega Excellence, Coconoil, Viridian)

$1/3$ cup vegetable glycerin (I use $1/4$ cup as glycerin can be a little too sweet)

1 teaspoon butterscotch extract

$1/2$ cup tahini or sunflower seed butter

2 teaspoons (10 ml) E-lyte Balanced Electrolyte Concentrate

1 cup egg protein powder

$1/2$ cup organic whole flaxseed

1 cup organic sesame seeds

$11/2$ cups pecans, ground

$1/2$ cup pecans, chopped

Melt the coconut butter over low heat. Remove it from the heat and add the remaining wet ingredients. Whisk until well blended. Combine the dry ingredients. Pour the wet ingredients into the dry and mix thoroughly.

Line a 9 by 9-inch baking pan with parchment paper and grease the pan with olive or coconut oil. Press the mix into the pan. Score into 12 bars and refrigerate to set.

Chocolate Hazelnut Power Bars

YIELD: 12 BARS

5 ounces cocoa butter

$1/3$ cup vegetable glycerin

2 teaspoons hazelnut extract (optional)

$1/2$ cup tahini or sunflower seed spread

1 teaspoon E-lyte Balanced Electrolyte Concentrate

1 cup walnuts

1 cup egg protein powder

$1/2$ cup raw cocoa

$1/2$ cup whole organic flaxseed

1 cup organic sesame seeds

Melt the cocoa butter over low heat. Remove from the heat and blend it with the other wet ingredients. Grind the walnuts and combine them with the other dry ingredients. Pour the wet ingredients into the dry and mix thoroughly.

Line a 9 by 9-inch baking pan with parchment paper and grease the pan with olive or coconut oil. Press the mix into the pan. Score into 12 bars and refrigerate to set.

LUNCHES OR EVENING MEALS

Quinoa Tabbouleh

This recipe is not strictly high-fat low-carb, but it's heavy on the parsley, which is rich in PQQ, the only new essential nutrient to be discovered in the last half-century. It stimulates the production of new mitochondria, the tiny energy-producing batteries in every cell. And it's delicious.

1 cup quinoa, uncooked

$1^1/_2$ cups fresh flat-leaved parsley (a mix of curly and flat-leaved gives more texture)

$^3/_4$ cup fresh mint

2 fresh tomatoes

$^1/_4$ cup spring onions, finely chopped

$^1/_4$ cup extra-virgin olive oil

$^1/_4$ cup freshly squeezed lemon juice

2 kale leaves

1 head bok choy

Spices

1 tablespoon finely ground black pepper

1 tablespoon ground allspice

1 tablespoon ground cinnamon

1 teaspoon grated nutmeg

1 teaspoon ground coriander

1 teaspoon ground cloves

1 teaspoon ground ginger

Wash the quinoa in a fine mesh sieve until the water runs clear, and drain.

Spread the quinoa in a skillet. Turn the heat to medium and let the quinoa heat until the moisture is gone. (You can skip this step if you are using the spices.) Continue to heat the quinoa for 15 minutes or until it smells toasty and fragrant. Remove from the heat when it is golden-brown and popping.

Place the quinoa in a saucepan with two cups of water and the spices, and bring to a boil. Reduce to a simmer and cover the pan. Cook for 10–15 minutes, stir, and let cool to room temperature.

Add all the vegetables and herbs and mix well. Dice the tomatoes and remove any excess seeds and liquid. Mix the olive oil and lemon in a separate bowl. Stir this into the salad and mix well.

Serve with poached trout or wild salmon.

GALLBLADDER-RELIEF RECIPES

(With grateful thanks to Deborah Graefer
of www.gallbladderattack.com)

Beet Recipe

This recipe is helpful for treatment of gallbladder pain.

1 large organic beet or raw beetroot, washed,
coarsely grated (not peeled unless not organic)

Lemon juice to taste (about $1/4$ lemon)

1 to 2 tablespoons flaxseed oil (flaxseed oil is by far the superior
choice here, as it is an omega-3 essential fatty acid, but use olive
oil if you are insulin resistant)

Take 1 teaspoon of this mixture every hour throughout the
day. On day two and three make a fresh batch, using $1/4$ of
a large beet. Take 1 teaspoon of mixture 3 to 4 times a day
or more often.

Make this mixture frequently to add to your salads or to
eat alone, as above, 2 or 3 times a week. This will keep the
bile thin and moving.

Notes: If you cannot get organic beets, be sure to peel them.
Otherwise, use the peel as well.

Eat your regular meals throughout this period, striving to
eat lots of fresh vegetables, good fats, and avoiding refined
sugars and processed foods.

Green Soup Recipe for Relief
of Gallbladder Pain

(The following two recipes thanks to Debbie Graefer
of gallbladderattack.com)

*Please note that **this soup is really an everyday soup that can help with the
associated general sluggishness and niggly aches and pains. It is not for a
gallbladder colic attack!** What we mean by this is that this is an everyday
soup that should help with bile flow and those low-grade aches and pains
of everyday gallbladder malfunction. If you are suffering with a full-blown
gallbladder attack use phosphoric acid drops or the Flaxseed Tea recipe
(below). Liquids are best during an attack. You could try the Beet Recipe
(previous); many find it helps, but others do better with just liquids.
This recipe is wonderful for relief from all sorts of gastric disturbances
such as stomach pain, gas, and indigestion. I do not add any fat or salt to
this recipe. It can be used anytime but is particularly useful as a three-day
fast with nothing else but water. It is both nourishing and easy to digest.
You can alter the amounts to taste. More beans add more sweetness.*

One bunch parsley, coarsely chopped

3 medium zucchini, thickly sliced

$1/2$ pound green beans

5 stalks celery, thickly sliced

Steam together for 8 to 10 minutes, or partially steam and
boil in $1/2$ cup water. You will retain more nutrients and flavor if you use a steamer. Purée in a blender.

(*Adopted from the recipe from Dr. Henry Beiler.*)

Flaxseed Tea

Useful during a gallbladder attack.

1 tablespoon organic flaxseeds

$2^1/2$ cups water

Boil the flaxseeds in the water for 5 minutes. Steep 10 minutes. Strain and sip slowly.

AT-HOME GENERAL GALLBLADDER SUPPORT

While we are on the topic of the good old gallbladder, it can be a huge problem—especially for some of us who fit that category of fair, fat, forty, female, and fertile. We spend an awful lot of time helping support gallbladders in our clinic so we felt it would be a good idea to share some things that work and that you can do at home.

Bitter Foods and Herbs

Here is our first little gem: bitter herbs. These are really bitter foods, and the beauty of bitter foods is that they stimulate the vagus nerve on the tongue, which triggers the release of digestive juices farther down in the digestive tract. They promote the production and secretion of bile, helping to keep it moving through your liver and gallbladder. Swedish bitters is a brand you have probably heard of; this needs to be consumed before meals. Bitter foods include beet leaves, dandelion leaves, chicory leaves, endive, radicchio, beets, mint leaves, globe artichoke, radish, lemons, limes, arugula (rocket), kale, watercress, basil, and cabbage. Try to include these fruits and vegetables in your diet daily to ensure you clean up your gallbladder.

There are also a few foods well known to upset the gallbladder, so you should remove these from your diet when possible. The worst offenders are gluten, sugar, pork, eggs, onions, and dairy products. A2 milk, (a cow's milk containing a less-common form of casein, available in the United Kingdom, Australia, and New Zealand), isn't any better. You can also add chocolate to this list. You should be able to return to eating pork and eggs fairly soon in small amounts once you are feeling better, but the others are best eliminated. Also, you may be told to stop any fat and oil consumption. While this is a bandage to stop all the pain it is a short-term solution. In the long-term this will do more harm than good because the gallbladder needs to contract and empty. If not, you are at risk of gallstone formation (assuming you are not reading this because you already have gallstones); you need good fats to help with the inflammation and contraction of the gallbladder. Ensure that you have plenty of good fats such as organic extra-virgin olive oil, macadamia oil, avocado oil, and our dearest food friend, cold-pressed coconut oil, and avoid the foods on the list above.

SUPPLEMENTS AND GALLSTONE RELIEF PROGRAM

There are a few supplements—just a handful—that you would do well to take for any problem anywhere in the digestive system. We would look you in the eye and tell you, "You cannot harm yourself by taking these in the way we recommend here." It is not true that all nutrients are completely safe; after all, you could kill yourself with too much water. You would have to work at it, mind you, and that's true for most nutrients as well—more so than for most medicines. You can get minor but disagreeable side effects from them, such as nausea or abdominal discomfort, particularly if you start with too much. Always start with a small dose and build up gradually, giving your digestion time to adapt.

There is also a list of supplements that are specific to each part of the digestion, dealt with further down, but let's start with the big four.

A. THE FOUR UNIVERSAL SUPPLEMENTS

1. Vitamin D

Treatment dose: 10,000 International Units (IU) daily, for no more than three months

Maintenance dose: 5,000 IU daily

Form: must be vitamin D_3 (cholecalciferol), not D_2 (ergocalciferol)

Best taken: with a meal containing protein and/or oil/fat, for best absorption. Mix it into the food or, better still, into a drink such as those suggested in the previous section. This will spread it around to as much of the bowel as possible.

Vitamin D is really a steroid hormone like cortisol, estrogen, or testosterone. It is only considered a vitamin (a molecule that is *vital* to obtain in food) because we usually don't get it the way we were meant to, from sunlight hitting our skin. Now, if you live in Southern California, you have access to a lot more sunlight than if you live in the Northeast United States, but unless you hang out at the beach a lot you probably don't take advantage of it. Most of us only see the sun when walking from our house to the car or from the subway to our office. That's why most people, everywhere, are deficient in vitamin D. In many studies all over the world, the only group that consistently had adequate vitamin D levels were Israeli lifeguards—people with European skin out all day in a very sunny place. People at the opposite end of the spectrum—with Afro-Caribbean coloring living in, let's say, New York, are highly likely to be low on the "sunshine vitamin." That has to be why the African guy mentioned in the case in Chapter 9 improved so rapidly and dramatically.

So we can start by assuming that you're low on vitamin D. In any case, it's hard to overdose on it—possible, but really hard. To my knowledge it has only ever happened when manufacturers have seriously messed up on the number of zeros in the dose they put into something. It won't happen because you take a few extra pills.

We know that vitamin D protects against a number of cancers, and, in fact, colon cancer was the first to be figured out. We are now starting to understand how it does this, and it has to do with the junctions between cells that we discussed in the Leaky Gut chapter. If you are low in vitamin D these junctions are less effective, the communication between cells that keeps them well-behaved is reduced, and the risk of them going "rogue" is increased.

These junctions are also important in the digestive tract to keep the gut contents from leaking out, and, when you are vitamin D deficient, those junctions are not repaired after an injury.[1] Just one dose of aspirin could cause what amounts to an injury, setting off one of those self-perpetuating cycles of inflammation. So you really need enough vitamin D to repair the gut lining.

Vitamin D also helps to protect you against viral and other infections. Keeping in mind what a bout of flu can do to your gut lining, isn't it wise to stay topped up on this nutrient?

Vitamin D has a synergistic effect with vitamin C. Research suggests that you may get benefit from a combination of vitamins D and C that you don't get from either of them alone.[2] The study looked at free-radical damage (oxidative stress), which is part of every type of inflammation. The two vitamins together improved every marker for injury.

2. Vitamin C

Treatment dose: bowel tolerance dose—see inset

Maintenance dose: 2–4 grams (g) ($1/2$ to 1 teaspoon of powder) daily, in water

Form: dissolved powder is better than capsules, which are better than tablets. If it irritates (it is a weak acid, after all), use a buffered form or mix it fifty-fifty with bicarbonate. Be careful, it will fizz.

Best taken: sufficiently diluted, in frequent small doses throughout the day.

Another nutrient that we are generally deficient in, but for different reasons, is vitamin C. Humans, unlike most creatures, cannot make vitamin C in our bodies, so we have to get it from food. But we often don't manage or don't bother, and these days we are exposed to so many different toxins that we probably need more than our ancestors did.

Vitamin C—also known as ascorbic acid — is important for the gut in a number of ways:

• It is a major antioxidant, protecting against free radical damage from all sorts of toxins.

• Your immune system uses it when fighting infections.

• It is the body's natural antihistamine, preventing inflammation from getting out of hand.

• It is necessary for the production of collagen, the connective tissue that effectively holds us together. Defective collagen causes the bruising, bleeding, and failed wound-healing in scurvy (a severe vitamin C deficiency).

As you get healthier, the useful life span of ascorbate inside your body will increase and less will be needed to achieve the desired effect. Then you can reduce your intake; indeed, you will need to, as less will be needed to produce watery bowel motions.

Dissolving vitamin C in a larger quantity of liquid may be easier than making up a small batch every time. Use a sealable bottle such as a mineral water bottle. Dissolved ascorbate is stable for a day, but no longer, if it is kept in a sealed bottle under refrigeration when possible.

TITRATING VITAMIN C TO BOWEL TOLERANCE

This is a way to achieve the maximum intake of ascorbic acid without side effects like diarrhea, which only happens when your body can't absorb any more vitamin C.

First, dissolve 2 g ($^1/_2$ teaspoon) of vitamin C powder (ascorbic acid or buffered ascorbate) in 2 fluid ounces (oz) of water or juice. Drink the liquid. Repeat this every thirty minutes until watery bowel motions occur (as if you had taken an enema). If watery bowel motions have not occurred after a full day of this, begin again in the morning, this time at one level teaspoonful (4 g) in 2 oz of water or juice every fifteen minutes. When watery bowel motions occur, stop consuming the ascorbate for that day.

Next, calculate the total ascorbate consumed during the day. For example, 2 g x 12 doses = 24 g. Or 4 g x 22 doses = 88 g. Whatever the total dose, your approximate daily need ("bowel tolerance") is around three-quarters of this level. Consume this as liquid, tablets, or capsules, in four or more doses per day. The aim is to achieve a consistent level of vitamin C in your bloodstream.

3. Zinc

Treatment dose: 30–50 mg daily

Maintenance dose: 10–15 mg

Form: reject zinc oxide or zinc carbonate; the basic form is zinc sulphate

Best taken: for some people, only a bedtime dose of zinc seems to work because it doesn't have to compete with phytates in your grains and nuts, but for others a mealtime dose is good. Try mealtime first because it sometimes causes nausea on an empty stomach.

Zinc is a trace element: in other words, a micronutrient—meaning there is not much of it in your body. In fact, there is no more than a teaspoonful, but it is needed inside every single cell. We are still not

ZINC TASTE TEST

Equipment: zinc sulphate in a 0.1 percent solution (there are various brands available)

Do the test well away from food or drink. Obviously, smoking interferes.

Hold a tablespoon of the solution in your mouth for 15 to 20 seconds, then swallow.

What you are looking for is a metallic taste, though some people report it as bitter or acidic, or dry, even rarely as sweet. Record your response using the following rating scale:

0 = no taste at all

1 = mild taste of something, developing only gradually

2 = taste of something, developing within a few seconds

3 = immediate taste

4 = immediate strong unpleasant taste

A result of 4 means you are not short of zinc, while 0 means you are very deficient.

sure how many enzymes in the body need zinc—certainly hundreds. Probably the most important single thing to remember about zinc is that, every time a gene is switched on, expressed, and makes a protein, the process needs zinc. That is why a lack of zinc affects growth and development and impairs wound healing. That also makes it very important for the gut, which has the fastest turnover of tissue in the body. The immune system also has to produce cells rapidly—when you need white blood cells you need them *now*—so immunity depends on zinc.

The ability to taste food depends on zinc because an important enzyme in saliva needs it. Back in the 1980s Derek Bryce-Smith worked out that if you are zinc-deficient you can't taste zinc, and to fix that you need a zinc drink! It is easy to test yourself, and you can follow the progress of your self-treatment too.

There can be other causes of loss of taste (ageusia or hypogeusia), but zinc deficiency will certainly cause it. The test is only a rough and ready one, but it's a useful guideline.[3]

4. Electrolytes

Treatment dose: up to 6 teaspoons daily

Maintenance dose: 1 to 2 teaspoons daily

Form: the E-lyte brand that we use contains (per teaspoon) approximately: 120 milligrams (mg) potassium, 60 mg sodium, and 40 mg magnesium. Several other similar brands are available.

Best taken: as liquid, mixed in water. Avoid any products containing sugar or sweeteners, and do not mix into sweetened drinks.

Every cell requires electrolytes to function. Sodium, potassium, magnesium, chloride, and phosphate are the main ones. When anything goes wrong in the digestion you are likely to develop an imbalance of these by losing them in loose bowel motions or vomiting, of course, but also from not eating and drinking well, or from not absorbing the nutrients you do eat.

You can also lose electrolytes in sweat, particularly when you exercise, which is why people take "sports drinks" to replace them. If you have ever suffered sunstroke you will know that it is deceptively easy to lose electrolytes in sweat. The only problem with these commercial remedies, as with diarrhea mixtures, is that they are loaded with sugar.

If you have a digestive disorder, electrolyte supplements will replace those you lose, which are needed by the cells of the gut just as much as, and maybe more than, other cells.

B. SUPPLEMENTS FOR DIGESTIVE SUPPORT

The next four supplements are all replacement therapies; they substitute for the juices or enzymes that, we suspect, your body is not making properly. It is difficult to get a test that will tell us precisely what is lacking from your system, so we usually have to figure out what helps by trial and error, and which, presumably, was therefore lacking.

You don't have to try these in the order they are set down here; this is just the sequence in which they are produced in the body. If there is no reason to do otherwise, we usually suggest starting with the pancreatic enzymes, which are the most all-purpose of these supplements.

You cannot know, at the beginning of treatment, how long you will have to take digestive supplements. For some it may be lifelong, but others will start to normalize the production of hydrochloric acid and digestive enzymes as their general health improves. Our advice is this:

- If at the end of three months you cannot be sure that you have had any real benefit from them, stop taking them because there is no point continuing.

- If by the end of three months you have definitely had a good benefit from them, try doing without them because you don't want to end up dependent.

- If at any stage you get unpleasant effects or symptoms that are not covered here, stop taking them immediately.

Betaine Hydrochloride

Treatment dose: 1 to 3 capsules per meal, depending on size of meal

Maintenance dose: same or less

Form: capsules, usually 600–650 mg each. If capsule dose is less take more to receive a full dose.

Best taken: before food, somewhere between fifteen to twenty minutes before and with the first mouthful

When these capsules dissolve in the stomach they release hydrochloric acid, which is what a healthy stomach produces.

A simple safety check first—because it is always possible that your stomach is producing too much hydrochloric acid, which can cause exactly the same symptoms as too little acid, possible, that is, but not probable. Although many doctors think that too much acid is the commonest cause of such symptoms, in fact it is the reflux that does it, and you don't need excess acid in order for reflux to give you the symptoms. So please check first that you tolerate them without getting symptoms of burning or indigestion, in which case you should stop them immediately (and eat something for them to work on).

That done, the capsules need to be taken at the beginning of meals to work properly—sometime between fifteen minutes before eating and the first mouthful. Another piece of trial and error will figure out the best timing for you.

Take one capsule at the start of a good-sized meal one day and, as long as you don't experience burning or indigestion, take two capsules with a similar meal the next day. Provided you still have no adverse digestive effects, try three capsules with an equivalent meal on the third day.

If you get an improvement of digestive symptoms, the number of capsules causing this improvement is probably enough and that dose should be taken with each meal, e.g., if two capsules remove your previous symptoms of flatulence or indigestion, take two capsules at the start of each good-sized meal and one capsule at the start of a light meal. If you had no digestive symptoms to start with and still don't get adverse symptoms with the test doses suggested above, take one to three capsules at the start of each meal depending on meal size. If three capsules cause some adverse abdominal symptoms but one or two didn't, take one or two capsules at the start of each meal.

Sometimes people find that they need an additional dose halfway through a large meal; it is okay to do this occasionally if you need to.

Bicarbonate

Treatment dose: from $1/2$ teaspoon to 2 full teaspoons

Maintenance dose: $1/2$ to 1 teaspoon

Form: mixed bicarbonate powder

Best taken: between 20 and 90 minutes after a meal

Bicarbonate is one of the oldest morning-after indigestion treatments in the book, and it does work although in part by treating reflux (see earlier chapter) in the esophagus rather than anything pancreatic. It needs to be taken after you finish eating so that you don't cancel the acid phase of digestion in the stomach or the stimulus to your own pancreas when the stomach contents hit the duodenum. This is a simple, easy, safe treatment that will also help to damp down food intolerance reactions.

If you have bloating symptoms after meals, try starting with half a level teaspoonful of bicarbonate of soda in a glass of water, any-where from twenty minutes after a meal to ninety minutes after. It's best to experiment and find your own dosage (see above) and timing. This will neutralize the acid from the stomach and activate your own pancreatic enzymes. Sometimes it also helps to activate the previous two supplements.

If bicarbonate helps the symptoms, you should continue to take it, but, because ordinary soda bicarbonate is entirely sodium-based, you don't want to take it long-term or you might risk blood pressure effects. Switch to a mixed bicarbonate product, which you can obtain from a health-food store.

Bile Salts

Treatment dose: 1 to 3 capsules

Maintenance dose: same

Form: capsules

Best taken: at the end of a meal, or even 20 minutes afterwards

The food component that is most laborious to digest is the fats; as well as the secretions of the stomach and pancreas. It needs the bile, and particularly the bile salts, whose purpose is to emulsify fats, breaking them up into smaller and smaller droplets, eventually called micelles, that the lipase enzyme can work on more effectively. If for whatever reason you do not produce enough bile yourself, it can be helpful to take capsules of bile salts.

Pancreatic Enzymes

Treatment dose: 1 to 3 capsules

Maintenance dose: same

Form: capsules (much better than tablets)

Best taken: from 15 minutes before a meal to 20 minutes after

Human and animal enzymes are designed to work in the bicarbonate-rich alkaline environment of the intestines, and not in the acidic stomach. When all we could get were enzymes derived from animals they had to be taken just after eating or they would get inactivated. Nowadays most digestive enzymes are plant enzymes and are not destroyed by stomach acid. This is why they can be taken at the beginning of a meal, and many people find them more beneficial if they are taken then.

Be prepared to establish by trial and error what timing suits you best; it could be anywhere between fifteen minutes before a meal to twenty minutes after finishing. You should not need more than one capsule for a small breakfast-type meal, two for a larger, more substantial one, and at the very most three for a big, lavish dinner. Many people find that just one capsule, before a meal that contains foods they know are problematic, is quite sufficient. It is easy to carry a few in your handbag or pocket against emergencies. Side effects and reactions to these are rare, but if you should have any you should work with a doctor or therapist.

C. HEALING THE GUT

In this section we are reaching the limits of what you can do for yourself, and in some instances you will need the help of a practitioner. For example, if you have persistent abdominal bloating or heaviness that does not seem to respond to anything we have suggested, you might come to suspect that you have an intestinal parasite. You can't treat that on your own for at least four reasons:

- The stool test for parasites needs a referral from a professional

- The drugs normally used these days, if you choose to follow that route, have to be prescribed by a doctor

- Some of the drugs are potentially quite toxic, and you will need monitoring

- It is always difficult to get a perspective on things from inside them

When healing the gut there is an old saying we mentioned earlier that's very relevant. It goes like this: "When you find you're in a hole, the first thing to do is stop digging." In other words, first find out what is harming the gut and get rid of it. Think about these factors:

- **Alcohol and NSAIDs:** Both alcoholic drinks and the nonsteroidal anti-inflammatory drugs strip the mucus and increase gut permeability with just one dose. That's aspirin, indomethacin, ibuprofen (Advil), celecoxib, all of them. Some are better than others, but none are completely safe. Cut them out.

- **Infections:** It's not the first thing you think of, unless you recently had an acute episode of diarrhea or vomiting or both, but it's certainly possible. You will need a practitioner to set up testing and treatment, though.

- **Food Intolerances:** See the previous Action Plan section for instructions on cutting out the big ones, wheat and dairy. Having gotten rid of these harmful agents, you can put together a relatively easy treatment regime with the following components.

Zinc-Carnosine

Treatment dose: approximately 40 mg twice daily

Maintenance dose: none

Form: capsules

Best taken: unknown

We have always known that zinc helps wound-healing (see The Four Universal Supplements at the beginning of this Action Section) and carnosine is well-known as an antioxidant and liver protectant. We now know that a compound of the two—meaning they are chemically bound together, not just the powders mixed up—has much more effect than the sum of its parts. For instance, zinc-carnosine can completely block the increased permeability caused by NSAIDs (of course you have to be smart or lucky enough to take it first). In experiments it also reduces stress ulcers and the fibrosis (scarring) that happens in NASH (non-alcoholic steato-hepatitis—fatty liver). Whatever the cause of an inflamed, leaky gut, it is likely to help.[4]

Glutamine

Treatment dose: 10 grams 3 times daily

Maintenance dose: none

Form: powder, dissolved or mixed into liquid

Best taken: away from food

Glutamine is the commonest amino acid in food. You would think that we got enough that way, but it has specific benefits when taken as a purified supplement.[5] If you are fed intravenously it does not take long for the small intestine to start to atrophy (shrivel) and become leaky, and then for gut bacteria, which are not necessarily "friendly," to get into the bloodstream. Glutamine by mouth, on its own, can repair all of that, which makes it a pretty powerful agent.[6] Its one drawback is the very large quantities you need to take, but at least it's tasteless.

Slippery Elm

Treatment dose: as tea: pour 2 cups boiling water over 4 g of powdered bark, then steep for 3–5 minutes. Drink 3 times daily. As capsules: 400–500 mg 3 times daily. As tincture: 5 ml 3 times daily (note: the tincture contains alcohol, which can be off-gassed by leaving it in a glass in a warm place for 10–20 minutes.

Maintenance dose: none

Form: various; see under Treatment Dose

Best taken: take 2 hours away from other herbs and supplements

Slippery elm is a herbal remedy with a number of uses. It contains mucilage that turns into a thick gel when mixed with water. It contains anti-oxidants that help to relieve inflammation in the bowel.[7] In addition, it helps to stimulate the nerve endings of the digestive tract so that mucus is increased. It you remember, linseed and chia seeds are similar in nature. You can purchase slippery elm in capsules, lozenges, and powder, the latter being the most common.[8]

Aloe Vera

Treatment dose: 100–200 mg daily

Maintenance dose: 100 mg

Form: liquid gel

Best taken: at night

Aloe is an old remedy for digestive and skin conditions that man has used for over 200 years. It is said to cleanse the digestive tract. It is a well-known topical remedy for burns, so it makes sense that it also stops that burning intestine feeling. It is part of the lily family, with different parts of the plant (the inner gel and/or the whole leaf) used for different reasons.

D. SPECIFIC DISORDERS

While much of the time the general rule works and you can apply certain supplements for a health issue anywhere in the digestive tract, sometimes we need to be more specific or target the organ directly. We have categorized some of the more specific supplement options below.

ORAL HEALTH—GENERAL

Canker Sores

Treatment: Deglycerized licorice

Treatment dose: 380 mg 1 to 2 times daily

Maintenance dose: not applicable

Form: chewable tablets

Best taken: 20 minutes before meals

Deglycerized licorice (DGL) has anti-inflammatory,[9] antiviral,[10] and anti-allergic properties. DGL accelerates growth and regeneration in mucosal cells. Clinicians have used it for many years to heal digestive conditions such as reflux, ulcers,[11] and respiratory disease.

Periodontal Disease

Treatment: Coenzyme Q_{10} (CoQ_{10})

Treatment dose: 150–300 mg daily

Maintenance dose: 150 mg

Form: Ubiquinol capsules

Best taken: with oily or fatty foods

CoQ_{10} is notably known for its role in energy production in the power-houses of our cells. It increases the supply of oxygen to the tissues. In a review of seven Japanese studies, 332 patients with periodontal disease were followed up and 70 percent showed significant improvement in periodontal disease by supplementing with CoQ_{10}. Because it is fat-soluble it easily moves into the tissues, but as we age the amount we make diminishes significantly so some say we should all take this supplement after the age of forty-five. Due to the direct link between heart disease and poor gum health we should be taking more care of our gums.[12]

Other options for periodontal disease include baseline nutrients such as protein and vitamin A.

Vitamin B-Complex

The B vitamins are necessary to improve protein synthesis to aid with healing and repair. They also help prevent the breakdown of the mucosal barrier in response to bacterial activity. The elderly, vegans (who may not eat enough B_{12}), patients who take medications such as H_2 blockers (acid reducers), phenytoin, and methotrexate need to add B vitamin supplements to their diet. We all need B vitamins for energy, so we advise that more green leafy vegetables, meat, and dairy would be great additions to your daily regime. There are many B vitamin complexes available, all with a slightly different focus.

Treatment dose: High strength, 1 per day one month

Maintenance dose: Low strength

Form: Preferably enzyme activates forms of B vitamins

Best taken: With breakfast, and lunch if needed twice. High dose B_6 can induce vivid dreams so you may wish to avoid B vitamins later in the day.

Vitamin E

People with poor gastrointestinal function, who are known to have difficulty absorbing nutrients, often run low on vitamin E. Being low on this antioxidant vitamin reduces antibody production and overall immune response, which is not good if you have bacteria living in and around the gum line. If you know you are one of these individuals, extra nuts, seeds, and their oils are a must to include in your diet.

Treatment dose: 400 IU daily

Form: Must contain tochopherols and tocotrienols

Best taken: with oils or fats as this is fat soluble. Add it to the neuro-lipid cocktail.

Vitamin K

Vitamin K is a guy who really keeps himself under wraps most of the time. It is seriously overshadowed by calcium but equally as important for bone density and strength, and of course good tooth formation and anchorage of the teeth into the jaw. If you are taking anticoagulant therapy you need to ask your regular doctor if you can take vitamin K. If not you can get it from green leafy vegetables, liver, and legumes.

Treatment dose: 200 mcg per day

Form: K2

Best taken: with good fats/oils. Also this vitamin works in synergy with vitamin D_3 so consider a combined product, especially if you have infection and bone loss.

Boron

Keep eating those green leafy vegetables and legumes for their boron content. Again, this trace mineral is needed in tiny amounts, but it helps calcium balance. You might see signs of impaired wound and gum healing if you need this, but a good bone-support supplement might be the easiest way to obtain this.

Treatment dose: 750 mcg per day

Form: as chelate. Best taken as part of a bone supporting complex or a basic mineral complex.

Best taken: with food.

Calcium

You have all heard of calcium. We have been advised to drink plenty of milk to get enough of this wonderful mineral to help our teeth remain strong and firmly rooted in their sockets. To be honest, there isn't much point in just taking calcium by itself because it requires the synergy of all the other trace minerals and supporting vitamins to ensure it gets to where it needs to be. If you are a young woman or postmenopausal then your need might be greater. In addition to dairy, which isn't the most bioavailable source of calcium, tofu, legumes, nuts, and seeds are also good sources.

Treatment dose: 800 mg

Form: as chelate

Best taken: away from zinc and iron as they compete for absorption.

Copper

We hear about copper quite a bit in terms of copper bracelets for arthritis. Some people swear by these, but others just say their wrists turn green. I hope that doesn't happen to your insides, too. Joking aside, copper has to be balanced with zinc in a 1:10 ratio because copper is antagonistic to zinc. Most of us have a high requirement for zinc when our digestion is not as good as we would like, but copper is also important for its role in providing tensile strength to collagen and improving bone strength. It is also said to assist with neutrophil proliferation.

Treatment dose: 900 mcg per day

Forms: should be taken in a ratio of 1:10 with zinc

Best taken: with zinc. Should not be taken as a single supplement unless it is monitored by a practitioner.

Iron

Iron (Fe) is a strange mineral. Women need it a fair amount during their child-bearing years due to the menses, but that need diminishes somewhat postmenopause. Iron is very important for immune building; the phagocytic activity of the neutrophils is enhanced with good levels of iron. It also encourages those lymphocytes to grow and, where bacteria reside, we need all the white cells the body can make available. If you are a regular antacid user you should be aware that you have an increased need for iron. Adequate levels can be obtained from red meat and eggs as long as you are digesting and absorbing fully.

Treatment dose: 8 mgs daily

Forms: as ferrous gluconate or fumarate. Ferrous sulphate can cause digestive upset.

Taken: with vitamin C foods to help absorption and as part of a combined health complex.

Magnesium

The benefits of magnesium are far and wide. At a very basic level magnesium really helps constipation, but for our purposes it helps the body manage calcium and electrolyte levels. (We have already seen how important those are.) You have to be careful of the version you take, as all magnesium isn't created equal. If you need to get a sluggish bowel going then magnesium citrate will work wonders but it can be an irritant to some. In those cases magnesium glycinate is much kinder and better absorbed.

Treatment dose: about 400 mg per day. Take to bowel tolerance (i.e., when loose stools occur, drop back by one tablet/capsule (100 mg).

Forms: amino acid chelates, malate, ascorbate

Taken: As capsules, powders, transdermal oils or sprays, magnesium baths. The best approach is to use both oral and transdermal.

GASTROESOPHAGEAL REFLUX DESEASE (GERD) AND HIATIS HERNIA SYNDROME/VAGUS NERVE IMBALANCE (HHS/VNI)

In addition to digestive support as necessary, some more specific remedies for this condition include zinc carnosine, DGL licorice, and phosphatidyl choline. See above for specifics on these treatments. Test and chelate for heavy metals with zinc and methionine (nickel) and selenium and methionine (for mercury) and/or glutathione. You must consult a practitioner to do this safely.

Treatment dose: one of each zinc and methionine before breakfast for two weeks, then one of each before breakfast and lunch for four weeks. Finally, back to one of each before breakfast for four more weeks.

Maintenance dose: none

Form: capsules

Best taken: on an empty stomach

Adding zinc to the chelation protocol is good for removing nickel from the system, while the adding selenium is good for mercury elimination.

Stress-Reducing Nutrients and Activities

Those suffering from GERD and HHS/VNI should make sure they provide complete digestive support to improve their condition. Primary support is provided by the four universal supplements—vitamins D and C, zinc, and electrolytes—described above. Secondary support is provided by the digestive support nutrients, herbs, and behaviors.

Breathing exercises and programs such as HeartMath® should be considered. Providing lower spine support, such as putting a roll behind the waist to retain the natural curvature of the spine (which stretches out the lower esophagus to reduce the incidence of a hiatus hernia sliding) can be valuable and is really important after eating.

Treatment: Vitamin B-Complex

Treatment dose: one per day with breakfast

Form: capsules

Best taken: with food

Treatment: Rhodioloa (roseroot)

Rhodioloa is an adaptogenic herb in that it helps the body adapt and fight stress.

Treatment dose: 1 or 2 per day with breakfast

Form: capsules

Best taken: with food

CANCER

No way can we tell you how to fix a cancer, any cancer, without the help of a good doctor. We won't even try. We certainly don't believe in simply rejecting surgery, chemotherapy, radiation, or other such treatments without good reason. What we do believe is this:

• Everybody is different, individual, and so is their cancer. There are no one-size-fits-all solutions.

• Nobody knows more about what you need than you do. Your voice must be heard when treatment decisions are being made.

- It's a percentages game. You get a few points advantage from one thing, a few from another; magic bullet treatments that just make it all go away are as rare as, well, magic bullets. So why would you not stack up all the points you can by using everything available? Surgery, chemotherapy, radiation, hormones, nutrition, lifestyle, mind power—they can each help, but they work so much better together. That's what is called integrative medicine.

If you have read through the previous chapters you will have noted that there are a number of things that cause or contribute to cancer; they mostly have to do with inflammation and/or irritation. Smoking is an obvious cause and so is too much alcohol. Persistent reflux is bad news for the esophagus; colitis increases your risk of colon cancer. These are all prevention issues, so you may think that once you have a cancer they are irrelevant, but you'd be wrong. They can influence how a cancer progresses and, anyway, getting a second cancer is not that unusual. So take care of all the commonsense stuff.

Apart from smoking, the most important thing to do for cancer is diet. You will find the diet you need in Action Plan, Section 1. There are two big reasons why the diet is important:

- Cancers love sugar; they depend on it and thrive on it. You, on the other hand, can get by without it.

- Cancers can starve you to death; you burn so much nutrition fighting them that you have to boost your diet to cope. You need *good* food.

GASTRIC ULCERS

In addition to digestive support (Action Plan, Section 1) and the top four (the beginning of Action Plan, Section 2) you may also wish to consider mastic gum.[13] There has been a stream of evidence in support of its activity in eradicating *Helicobacter pylori* and improving the mucous membrane of the gut.

Treatment: mastic gum

Treatment dose: 1 gm daily

Form: capsules

Best taken: twenty minutes before food

SMALL INTESTINAL BACTERIAL OVERGROWTH (SIBO)

SIBO can cause symptoms high up in the digestive tract or lower down in the colon. Some reflux symptoms originate in the small intestine.

Treatment: Oregano oil

Treatment dose: 200 mg 3 times daily for 6 weeks

Form: oil-based capsules

Best taken: away from probiotics

Oregano oil has a long-standing history of use in eradicating dysbiosis of many different forms.[14] It has also been used for infections of the mucous membranes in many organs. Please don't use oregano oil if you are pregnant.

Treatment: Garlic

Treatment dose: 600–1,200 mg daily in divided doses

Form: tablets

Best taken: with food

Allicin, the active component in garlic, has been studied for centuries. It has antifungal and antibacterial qualities that lend themselves beautifully to rebalancing gut bacteria.[15] You will need to be very careful if you have a lot of gut inflammation because garlic can irritate a sensitive gut. You also should not take garlic if you are taking anticoagulant medications such as warfarin. There seems to be a lot of inferior garlic preparations on the market, so be sure to find one with a high allicin content.

INFLAMMATORY BOWEL DISEASE

Diseases such as ulcerative colitis and Crohn's disease require quelling of the inflammation in addition to rebuilding of the protective mucous lining; phosphatidylcholine is a key player in the process.

Treatment: Phosphatidylcholine (PC)

Treatment dose: 1–2 tablespoons daily

Form: liquid or capsules

Best taken: in a power-based drink, such as our neurolipid cocktail, with omega-6 oils such as BodyBio Balance Oil in a ratio of 4(oil):1.

Phosphatidylcholine is undoubtedly the most important supplement for the gut, liver, and all cells of the body. PC helps cell membranes to stabilize, allowing transport of nutrients and electrolytes across the cell membranes and encouraging healing and repair. Please refer back to the information on PC in the chapter on the large bowel.

Treatment: Vitamin B_{12} (methylcobalamin)

Treatment dose: 1 mg per day for 4 weeks; then 1 mg per week for 4 weeks; then 1 mg per month

Form: sublingual tablets (dissolve under the tongue), oral spray, patches

Best taken: after food

B_{12} deficiency does not always present as anemia, but some weird neurological symptoms may present where there is obvious B_{12} deficiency. Numbness and tingling in the arms and legs is a classic symptom. Fatigue is another. In fact, many individuals with chronic fatigue struggle without regular B_{12}. The symptoms could take years to manifest due to the fact that we store B_{12} so it takes a very long time to run down our internal stores.

Treatment: Folate

Treatment dose: 1 mg daily for 1–4 months

Form: tablets

Best taken: with food

Folate deficiency is frequently seen in both ulcerative colitis (UC) and Crohn's disease (CD). B_{12} and folate are synergistic, in that a deficiency of one can be masked by a high intake of the other. For this reason they should be taken together. In fact, considering that around 40 percent of individuals are said to have a deficiency in the enzyme required to convert folate into a usable form for the body, the enzyme-activated form methyltetrahydrolfolate (MTHF) is the best one to try.

GALLSTONES

The following vitamins, botanicals, and supplements are all useful for treatment of gallstones. See the gallstone programs below. Program 1 would be followed for 6–12 days, then move on to Program 2.

Treatment: Vitamin E

Treatment dose: 200–400 International Units (IU) one per day

Use: primarily helps to prevent fat oxidization and rancidity. Must be taken in mixed tocopherols/tocotrienols form.

Treatment: Phosphatidylcholine

Treatment dose: 100 mg three times per day

Use: helps restoration of cell membranes and cell-to-cell communication, and helps to protect the liver.

Treatment: Fiber supplements: psyllium, glucomannan, pectin, oat bran

Treatment dose: minimum 5 gm per day

Use: fiber helps to maintain good bowel habits, thereby assisting with toxin removal

Treatment: Bile acids

Treatment dose: 1,000–1,500 mg per day

Use: help to assimilate fats and fatty acids, thin down bile, and help bile flow.

Treatment: Peppermint oil enteric coated (EC)

Treatment dose: 360 mg three times per day, between meals

Use: peppermint oil is useful for dissolving stones

Treatment: Sylimarin (not milk thistle)

Treatment dose: 70–210 mg per day

Use: antioxidant protection for the liver

Treatment: Curcumin

Treatment dose: 100–200 mg three times per day

Use: antioxidant, anti-inflammatory to quell inflammation and pain

Treatment: Dandelion root

Treatment dose (daily): dried–4 g; fluid extract–4–8 ml (1:1 in water); solid extract–250–500 mg (4:1 in water)

Preliminary Preparation for the Gallstone Relief Program

Use this preliminary program for between 1 and 4 months to soften and reduce gallstones before embarking on a gallstone program.

Taurine and beet: 100 mg each in a combination pill, 4 per meal

Phosphatidylcholine: 440 mg capsule, 1 per meal

Vitamin B-complex: 2 per meal

Liver support: 1 capsule per meal

Gallstone Program 1

Follow for 6–12 days.

Orthophosphoric acid liquid: 1 full bottle in 4 oz tomato juice daily for 6–14 days

Taurine (100 mg) and beet (100 mg): 4–6 tablets per meal

Gallstone Program 2

Follow for 6–14 days.

Taurine (100 mg) and beet (100 mg): 6 tablets per meal

Phosphatidylcholine (300 mg): 3 capsules per meal

Vitamin B_6 (P-5-P form): 4 per meal

Magnesium: 6–12 tablets or more at bedtime; take to bowel tolerance.

Super Phosphozyme: 3 tablets per meal

Iodine (liquid): 30 drops per meal

References

Chapter 1. Are You Down in the Mouth?

1. Richter, J.E. "Oesophageal Motility Disorders." *Lancet* 358 (Sep 8, 2001): 823–8.

2. Chen, N., et al. "Vaccination for Preventing Postherpetic Neuralgia." *Cochrane Database Syst Rev 3* (Mar 16, 2011): CD007795.

3. McEwen, B.S. "Protective and Damaging Effects of Stress Mediators: Central Role of the Brain." *N Eng J Med* 338 (1998): 171–9.

4. Haase, H., E. Mocchegiani, L. Rink. "Correlation between Zinc Status and Immune Function in the Elderly." *Biogerontology* 7(5–6) (Oct-Dec 2006): 421–8.

5. Cazzola, P., P. Mazzanti, G. Bossi G. "In Vivo Modulating Effect of a Calf Thymus Acid Lysate on Human T Lymphocyte Subsets an CD4+CD8 Ratio in the Course of Different Diseases." *Current Theories Research* 42 (1987): 1011–7.

6. Nolkemper, S., et al. "Antiviral Effect of Aqueous Extracts from Species of the Lamiaceae Family against Herpes Simplex Virus Type 1 and Type 2 in Vitro." *Planta Med* 72(15) (Dec 2006):1378–82.

7. Garewal, H.S., S. Schantz. "Emerging Role of Beta-Carotene and Antioxidant Nutrients in Prevention of Oral Cancer." *Arch Otolaryngol Head Neck Surg* 121(2) (Feb 1995): 141–4. Ibraham, K., N. Zafarey, S. Zubery. "Vitamin A and Carotene Levels in Squamous Cell Carcinoma of Oral Cavity and Oropharynx." *Clin Oncol* 3 (1997): 203–7.

8. Pannell, R.S., D.M. Fleming, K.W. Cross. "The Incidence of Molluscum Contagiosum, Scabies and Lichen Planus." *Epidemiol Infect* 133(6) (Dec 2005): 985–91.

9. Esfahanian, V., M.S. Shamami, M.S. Shamami. "Relationship between Osteoporosis and Periodontal Disease: Review of the Literature." *J Dent* (Tehran) 9(4) (Aut 2012): 256–64.

10. Famili, P., J. Cauley, J.B. Suzuki, R. Weyant. "Longitudinal Study of Periodontal Disease and Edentulism with Rates of Bone Loss in Older Women." *J Periodontol* 76(1) (Jan 2005): 11–5.

11. Dietrich, T., et al. "Association between Serum Concentrations of 25-Hydroxyvitamin D3 and Periodontal Disease in the US Population." *Am J Clin Nutr* 80(1) (Jul 2004): 108–13.

Chapter 2. Reflux, aka GERD

1. Rochlitz, S. *Hiatal Hernia Syndrome/Vagus Nerve Imbalance: A Missing Link to Chronic Illness, Allergies and Other Problems,* 2012 (at www.wellatlast.com, accessed Jun 2014).

2. Stiennon, O.A. *The Longitudinal Muscle in Esophageal Disease.* Internet edition. 1995. http:// http://www.esophagushoncho.com/ (accessed June 2014).

3. Mower, D. "The Role of Hypochlorhydria in Nutrient Deficiencies and Its Relevance to Age Related Pathologies." *Nutr Practitioner* (Spring 2005): 1–16.

4. Benjamin, E.J., et al. "Impact of Atrial Fibrillation on the Risk of Death: The Framingham Heart Study." *Circulation* 98 (1998): 946–52.

5. Kassarjian, Z., R.M. Russell. "Hypochlorhydria: A Factor in Nutrition." *Annu Rev Nutr* 9 (1989): 271–85.

6. Kelly, G. "Hydrochloric Acid: Physiological Functions and Clinical Implications." *Alt Med Rev* 2(2) (1997): 116–27.

7. Lokk, J. "News and Views on Folate and Elderly Persons." *J Gerontol A Biol Sci Med Sci* 58(4) (Apr 2003): 354–61.

8. Chandra, R.K. "Nutrition and the Immune System: An Introduction." *Am J Clin Nutr* 66(2) (1997): 460S–463S

9. Morris Brown, L., et al. "Adenocarcinoma of the Esophagus: Role of Obesity and Diet." *JNCI J Nat Cancer Inst* 87(2) (1995): 104–9.

10. Chen, X., C.S. Yang. "Esophageal Adenocarcinoma: A Review and Perspectives on the Mechanism of Carcinogenesis and Chemoprevention." *Carcinogenesis."* 22 (Aug 2001): 1119–29.

Chapter 3. Ulcers and Helicobacter Pylori

1. Marshall, B. J., J.R. Warren. "Unidentified Curved Bacilli in the Stomach of Patients with Gastritis and Peptic Ulceration." *Lancet* 1(8390) (Jun 16, 1984): 1311–5.

2. Yi-Qi Du, et al. "Adjuvant Probiotics Improve the Eradication Effect of Triple Therapy for Helicobacter Pylori Infection." *World J Gastroenterol* 18(43) (Nov 21, 2012): 6302–7.

3. Sezikli, M., et al. "Oxidative Stress in Helicobacter Pylori Infection: Does Supplementation with vitamins C and E Increase the Eradication Rate?" *Helicobacter* 14(4) (Aug 2009):280–5.

4. Salem, E.M., et al. "Comparative Study of Nigella Sativa and Triple Therapy in Eradication of Helicobacter Pylori in Patients with Non-Ulcer Dyspepsia." *Saudi J Gastroenterol* 16(3) (Jul-Sep 2010): 207–14.

5. Coxib and traditional NSAID Trialists' (CNT) Collaboration. "Vascular and Upper Gastrointestinal Effects of Non-Steroidal Anti-Inflammatory Drugs: Meta-Analyses of Individual Participant Data from Randomised Trials." *Lancet* 382 (9894) (Aug 31, 2013): 769–79.

Chapter 4. The Liver

1. Braganza, J.M., et al. "Lipid-Peroxidation (Free-Radical-Oxidation) Products in Bile from Patients with Pancreatic Disease." *Lancet* 2(8346) (Aug 1983): 375–9.

2. Miller, T.C., J. Gerth. "Behind the Numbers: How Many People in the United States Die or Suffer Serious Harm from Acetaminophen Overdose? *ProPublica* (Sep 20, 2013). http://www.propublica.org/article/tylenol-mcneil-fda-behind-the-numbers (accessed June 2014).

3. Neustadt, J., S.R. Pieczenik. "Medication-Induced Mitochondrial Damage and Disease." *Mol Nutr Food Res* 52(7) (Jul 2008): 780–8.

4. Pérez-Guisado, J., A. Muñoz-Serrano. "The Effect of the Spanish Ketogenic Mediterranean Diet on Nonalcoholic Fatty Liver Disease: A Pilot Study." *J Med Food* 14(7–8) (Jul-Aug 2011): 677–80.

5. Shi, X., et al. [A Multi-Center Clinical Study of N-acetylcysteine on Chronic Hepatitis B]. *Zhonghua ganzangbing zazhi* = Chinese journal of hepatology 13(1), (2005): 20–3 [Chinese].

6. Bass, S., N. Zook. "Intravenous Acetylcysteine for Indications Other Than Acetaminophen Overdose." *Am J Health-Syst Pharm* 70(17) (Sep 1, 2013); 1496–501.

Chapter 5. The Biliary Tree

1. National Health Service. Institute for Innovation and Improvement. "Cholecystectomy (Removal of the Gall Bladder)." http://www.institute.nhs.uk/quality_and_value/high_volume_care/cholecystectomy_(removal_of_the_gall_bladder).html (accessed June 2014).

2. Ash, M. "Bile Acids Make You Live Longer: A New Understanding." *White paper researched leadership*. Nutri-Link Ltd, 2008.

3. Bertok, L. "Bile Acids and Endotoxins: Physico-Chemical Defense of the Body." *Orv Hetil* 140 (1) (Jan 3, 1999): 3–8. Review [article in Hungarian].

4. Moritz, A. *The Liver and Gallbladder Miracle Cleanse: An All-Natural, At-Home Flush to Purify and Rejuvenate Your Body*. Berkeley, CA: Ulysses Press, 2007.

5. Osman, M., et al. "Biliary Parasites." *Dig Surg* (1998): 287–96.

6. Gardner, A. "C-Section May Disrupt "Good" Bacteria in Babies." Web MD HealthDay. http://www.webmd.com/baby/news/20130211/c-section-formula-may-disrupt-good-gut-bacteria-in-babies (accessed June 2014).

7. Gualradi, F., G. Salvatore. "Effect of Breast and Formula Feeding on Gut Microbiota Shaping in Newborns." *Frontiers in Cellular and Infection Biology* 2 (2012): 94.

Chapter 6. The Pancreas

1. Fieker, A., J. Philpott, M. Armand. "Enzyme Replacement Therapy for Pancreatic Insufficiency: Present and Future." *Clin Exp Gastroenterol* 4 (2011): 55–73.

2. Braganza, J.M., J.E. Jolley, W.R. Lee. "Occupational Chemicals and Pancreatitis: A Link?" *Int J Pancreatol* 1(1) (May 1986): 9–19.

3. Burim, R.V., et al. "Polymorphisms in Glutathione S-Transferases GSTM1, GSTT1 and GSTP1 and Cytochromes P450 CYP2E1 and CYP1A1 and Susceptibility to Cirrhosis or Pancreatitis in Alcoholics." *Mutagenesis* 19(4) (Jul 2004): 291–8.

4. de la Mano, A.M., et al. "Cholecystokinin Blockade Alters the Systemic Immune Response in Rats with Acute Pancreatitis." *Int J Exp Pathol* 5(2) (Apr 2004): 75–84.

5. Jaworek, J., T. Brzozowski, S.J. Konturek. "Melatonin as an Organoprotector in the Stomach and the Pancreas." *J Pineal Res* 38(2) (Mar 2005): 73–83.

Chapter 7. Dysbiosis

1. Hopkins, M.J., R. Sharp, G.T. Macfarlane. "Variation in Human Intestinal Microbiota with Age." *Dig Liver Dis* 34(Suppl 2) (Sep 2002): S12–8.

2. Hopkins, M.J., R. Sharp, G.T. Macfarlane. "Changes in Predominant Bacterial Populations in Human Faeces with Age and with Chlostridium Difficile Infection." *J Med Microbiol* 51(5) (May 2002): 448–54.

3. McFarland, L.V. "Meta-Analysis of Probiotics for the Prevention of Associated Diarrhea and the Treatment of Clostridium Difficile Disease." *Am J of Gastroenterol* 101(4) (Apr 2006): 812–22.

4. Williams, C., K.E. McColl. "Review Article: Proton Pump Inhibitors and Bacterial Overgrowth." *Aliment Pharmacol Ther* 23(1) (Jan 2006): 3–10.

Chapter 8. Leaky Gut

1. Healthy.Net: Healthy People, Healthy Planet. "Leaky Gut Syndromes: Breaking the Vicious Cycle." Healthworld Online. www.healthy.net/Health/Article/Leaky_Gut_Syndromes_Breaking_the_Vicious_Cycle/425/1 (accessed July 2014).

2. Shan, M., et al. "Mucus Enhances Gut Homeostasis and Oral Tolerance by Delivering Immunoregulatory Signals." *Science* 342(6157) (Oct 2013): 447–53.

3. Galland, L., H. Lafferty. *Gastrointestinal Dysregulation: Connections to Chronic Disease.* Gig Harbor, WA: Institute for Functional Medicine, 2008.

4. Dewar, D., C. Ciclitira. "Clinical Features and Diagnosis of Celiac Disease" *Gastroenterology* 128 (4) (2005): S19–S24.

5. Hadjivassiliou, M., et al. "Is Cryptic Gluten Sensitivity an Important Cause of Neurological Illness?" *Lancet* 347 (1996): 369–71.

6. Jensen, C. S., et al. "Experimental Systemic Contact Dermatitis from Nickel: A Dose-Response Study." *Contact Dermatitis* 49(3) (2003): 124–2.

7. Williams, M., et al. "Metal and Silicate Particles Including Nanoparticles Are Present in Electronic Cigarette Cartomizer Fluid and Aerosol." *PloS One* 8(3) (Mar 20, 2013): e57987. doi:10.1371/journal.pone.0057987.

8. Cazzato, I.A., et al. "Lactose Intolerance in Systemic Nickel Allergy Syndrome." *Int J Immunopathol Pharmacol* 24(2) (Apr-Jun 2011): 535–7.

Chapter 9. The Large Intestine and Its Goings On or Out

1. Bollinger, R.R., et al. "Biofilms in the Large Bowel Suggest an Apparent Function of the Human Vermiform Appendix." *J Theor Biol* 249(4) (Dec 21, 2007): 826–31.

2. Clark, K.J., et al. "Determination of the Optimal Ratio of Linoleic Acid to Alpha-Linolenic Acid in Infant Formulas." *J Pediatr* 120(4 Pt 2) (Apr 1992): S151–8.

3. Segain, J.P., et al. "Butyrate Inhibits Inflammatory Responses through NFkB Inhibition: Implications for Crohn's Disease." *Gut* 47(3) (Sep 2000): 397–403.

4. Anderson, V., et al. "Diet and Risk of Inflammatory Bowel Disease." *Dig Liver Dis* 44(3) (Mar 2012): 185–94.

5. Romagnuolo, J., et al. "Hyperhomocysteinemia and Inflammatory Bowel Disease: Prevalence and Predictors in a Cross-Sectional Study." *Am J Gastroenterol* 96(7) (Jul 2001): 2143–9

6. Stremmel, W., et al., "Retarded Release PC Benefits Patients with Chronic Active Ulcerative Colitis." *Gut* 54(7) (2005): 996–71.

7. Lichtenberger, L.M., et al. "Non-Steroidal Anti-Inflammatory Drugs (NSAIDs) Associate with Zwitterionic Phospholipids: Insight into the Mechanism and Reversal of NSAID-Induced Gastrointestinal Injury." *Nat Med* 1(12) (Feb 1995): 154–8.

8. Gibson, P.R., J.G. Muir. "Reinforcing the Mucus: A New Therapeutic Approach for Ulcerative Colitis." *Gut* 54(7) (Jul 2005): 900–3.

9. Strate, L.L., et al. "Nut, Corn, and Popcorn Consumption and the Incidence of Diverticular Disease." *JAMA* 300(8) (Aug 27 2008): 907–14.

Action Plan, Section 1: Nutritional Approach

1. Zentek, J., et al. "Nutritional and Physiological Role of Medium-Chain Triglycerides and Medium-Chain Fatty Acids in Piglets." *Anim Health Res Rev* 12(1) (Jun 2011): 83–93.

2. Gamonski, W. "The True Potency of the Pumpkin Seed." *Life Extens* (Oct 2012): 95–8.

3. Anjum, F.M., et al. "Nutritional and Therapeutic Potential of Sunflower Seeds: A Review." *Brit Food J* 114(4) (2012): 544–52.

4. Mohd Ali, N., et al. "The Promising Future of Chia, *Salvia hispanica L.*" *J Biomed Biotech* 2012 (Epub Nov 21, 2012). doi:10.1155/2012/171956.

5. Ridges, L., et al. "Cholesterol Lowering Benefits of Soy and Linseed Enriched Foods." *Asia Pac J Clin Nutr* 10(3) (2001): 204–11.

6. Anilakumar, K., et al. "Nutritional, Medicinal and Industrial Uses of Sesame (*Sesamum indicum L.*) Seeds: An Overview." *Agriculturae Conspectus Scientificus* 75(4) (2010): 159–68.

7. Eder, C. "A Wealth of Health Found in Walnuts." *Life Extens* (Aug 2011): 1–4.

8. Howard, M. E., N.D. White. "Potential Benefits of Cinnamon in Type 2 Diabetes." *Amer J Lifestyle Med* 7 (2012): 23–6.

9. Haniadka, R., et al. "A Review of the Gastroprotective Effects of Ginger (*Zingiber officinale Roscoe*)." *Food Funct* 4(6) (Jun 2013): 845–55.

10. Rennard, B.O., et al. "Chicken Soup Inhibits Neutrophil Chemotaxis in Vitro." Chest 118(4) Oct 2000: 1150–57.

Action Plan, Section 2: Supplements and Gallstone Relief Program

1. Kong, J., Z. Zhang Z, et al. "Novel Role of the Vitamin D Receptor in Maintaining the Integrity of the Intestinal Mucosal Barrier." *Am J Physiol Gastrointest Liver Physiol* 294(1) (Jan 2008): G208–16.

2722223

2. Ekici, F., B. Ozyurt H. Erdogan. "The Combination of Vitamin D3 and Dehydroascorbic Acid Administration Attenuates Brain Damage in Focal Ischemia." *Neurol Sci* 30(3) (Jun 2009): 207–12.

3. Eaton, K., I. Betteley, M. Harris. "Diagnosing Human Zinc Deficiency. A Comparison between the Bryce-Smith Test and Sweat Mineral Analysis." *J Nutr Med* 1(2) (1990): 113–7.

4. Mahmood, A., et al. "Zinc Carnosine, A Health Food Supplement That Stabilises Small Bowel Integrity and Stimulates Gut Repair Processes." *Gut* 56(2) (Feb 2007): 168–75.

5. Noé, J.E. "L-Glutamine Use in the Treatment and Prevention of Mucositis and Cachexia: A Naturopathic Perspective." *Integr Cancer Ther* 8(4) (Dec 2009): 409–15.

6. Souba, W.W. "The Gut: A Key Metabolic Organ Following Surgical Stress: Benefits of Glutamine Supplementation." *Contem Surg* 35(5A) (1989): 5–13.

7. Bock, S. "Integrative Medical Treatment of Inflammatory Bowel Disease." *Int J Integr Med* 2(5) (2000): 21–9.

8. Langmead, L., et al. "Antioxidant Effects of Herbal Therapies Used by Patients with Inflammatory Bowel Disease: An In Vitro Study." *Aliment Pharmacol Ther* 16(2) (Feb 2001): 197–205.

9. Deniz, G., S.E. Christmas, P.M. Johnson. "Soluble Mediators and Cytokines Produced by Human CD3-Leucocyte Clones from Decidualized Endometrium." *Immunology* 87(1) (Jan 1996): 92–8.

10. Fiore, C., et al. "Antiviral Effects of Glycyrrhiza Species." *Phytother Res* 22(2) (Feb 2008): 141–8.

11. Morgan, A.G., C. Pacsoo, W.A. McAdam. "Maintenance Therapy: A Two Year Comparison between Caved-S and Cimetidine Treatment in the Prevention of Symptomatic Gastric Ulcer Recurrence." *Gut* 26(6) (June 1985): 599–602.

12. Tanzer, J.M., G.J. Hageage. "Polyphosphate Inhibition of Growth of Plaques Formed by Streptococci and Diphtheroids Implicated in Oral Disease." *Infect Immun* 1(6) (Jun 1970): 604–6.

13. Paraschos, S. "Chios Gum Mastic: A Review of Its Biological Activities." *Curr Med Chem* 19(14) (2012): 2292–302.

14. Force, M., W.S. Sparks, R.A. Ronzio. "Inhibition of Enteric Parasites by Emulsified Oil of Oregano In Vivo." *Phytother Res* 14(3) (May 2000): 213–4.

15. Chorlton, M., et al. "PTH-086 Investigation of the Antimicrobial Activity of Essential Oils of Culinary and Medicinal Herbs and Spices against Selected Gastrointestinal Pathogens." *Gut* 62 (Suppl 1) (2013): A246.

INDEX

Acetaminophen, 50, 51, 55, 82
  poisoning, 50–51
Achalasia, 33–34
Acid erosion, 19, 25
Action plans
  nutritional, 121–142
  supplemental, 143–164
Adenocarcinoma, 33
Adrenaline, 30
Aging, 60, 89
Albumin, 52
Alcohol, 22, 51, 55, 80, 81, 83, 84,
  99, 153, 162
ALD (alcoholic liver disease), 52
Allergens, 8, 101
Allergies, 98, 104, 125
Allicin, 163
Aloe vera, 155
Alpha 1 gliadin antibody assay, 9
Alpha-lipoic acid, 56, 84
Amino acids, 86, 154
Amylases, 4, 76
Analgesic withdrawal syndrome, 45
Anemia, 3, 79, 114, 116
Angiograms, 67
Anne's Linseed Bread, 136–137
Anne's Paleo Porridge, 134–135
Antacids, 39, 159
Antibiotics, 9, 42, 89–90, 92
Antihistamines, 146
Antioxidants, 56, 59, 84, 145, 155,
  157, 166
Antrum, 38
APAP. See Acetaminophen.
Appendix, 109
Apples, 129
Aphthous stomatitis. See Canker sores.

Arginine, 11
Arteries, hepatic, 48
Arthred, 126
Arthritis, 105
Aspirin, 44, 144
Asthma, 28
Atrial fibrillation, 31
Attention deficit hyperactivity
  disorder (ADHD), 28
Autism spectrum disorders, 112
Autodigestion, 80
Avocados, 129, 130

Bacillus thuringiensis (Bt), 99
Bacteria, 23, 40, 42, 60, 71, 78,
  87–91, 99, 110
Barrett's esophagus, 25, 33
Beans, green, 141
Beet Recipe, 140
Beetroot complex, 73
Beets, 166
Berries, 123
Beta-carotene, 12
Beta Plus, 73
Beta TCP, 73
Betaine, 59, 126
Betaine hydrochloride (HCl), 73,
  150–151
Beverages, carbonated, 22, 36, 124
Bicarbonate, 37–38, 41, 70, 76, 80,
  85, 126, 136, 151
Bile, 28, 29, 37, 38, 48, 49, 50,
  58–62, 69, 76, 85, 142
Bile acids, 19, 59, 60, 64, 165
Bile duct, 48, 49, 58, 63, 66, 75, 81
Bile salts, 49, 58, 60, 77, 126, 152
Biliary colic, 65

Biliary flukes, 62–63
Biliary tree, 57–73
Bilirubin, 49, 50, 55, 66
Biotin, 88
Bisphenol A (BPA), 64
Black Seed. *See Nigella sativa.*
Bleeding, 79
Blenders, 127, 129
Bloating, 29, 35–36, 78–79, 87, 151
Blood, 48, 59, 96
    clotting, 59, 60
Bok choy, 130
Bolus, food, 19, 69
Bones, 14, 59, 116, 131, 158, 159
Boron, 158
Bowel. *See Intestines, large.*
Bowel tolerance, 146, 160
Bread, 102, 105, 123, 136–137
Breakfast, 122, 134–136
Breathing exercises, 161
Broths, 131–132
Brush border, 86
Bryce-Smith, Derek, 148
Bulimia, 38
Burns, 155
Butter, 123, 137
Butterscotch, 137
Butterscotch Pecan Power Bars, 137
Butyrate, 56, 88, 115

Cadmium, 106
Caesarian births, 71–72, 88
Caffeine, 36, 84
Calcium, 14, 33, 59, 111, 114, 116,
    131, 158–159, 160
Campylobacter pylori. See
    Helicobacter pylori.
Canaliculi, 49
Cancers, 34–35, 144, 161–162
    bile duct/biliary tree, 63, 64, 66–68
    colon, 144, 162
    esophageal, 23, 25, 33–36, 162
    kidney, 105
    liver, 53
    oral, 12
    squamous cell, 33
    stomach, 40, 42

Candida albicans, 9
Candidiasis, 9–10
Canines, 6
Canker sores, 7–9
    supplement for, 156
Carbohydrates, 21, 36, 76, 96, 126
Cardiac sphincter. *See* Sphincters,
    cardiac.
Cardiovascular disease. *See* Heart
    disease.
Care pathways, 57
Casein, 8, 9, 142
Cashews, 106
CCK. *See* Cholecystokinin (CCK).
Cecum, 109
Celery, 129, 130, 141
Celiac disease, 8, 61–62, 82, 88,
    102–106
    genes and, 102
    tests for, 102
Celiac syndrome, 77, 78, 101
Cells, 5, 52, 60, 121–122, 134, 156,
    164, 165
    epithelial, 97, 104
    fat, 60
    goblet, 86
    intestinal, 87, 96, 98, 148
    nerve, 97
    T helper, 11
    white blood, 114, 131, 134, 159
Cheeses, 123
Chemotherapy, 34–35
Chewing, 1, 2, 4–5, 21
Chicken, 132
Chloride, 148
Chocolate, 22, 56, 106, 142
Chocolate Hazelnut Power Bars, 138
Cholangiocarcinoma. *See* Cancer, bile
    duct/biliary tree.
Cholangitis, 62, 66
Cholecystectomies, 57
Cholecystitis, 62, 65
Cholecystokinin (CCK), 28, 38, 58,
    61–62, 69, 76, 83, 84, 105
    feedback loop failure, 68–73
Cholesterol, 58–59, 63, 64, 86, 134
Cholestyramine, 60

Choline, 59
Chyme, 58, 69, 85, 111
Cigarettes, electronic, 107
Cimetidine, 39
Cinnamon, 135
Circulation, 59
Cirrhosis, 52, 53
Clostridium difficile, 72, 99
Clotting factors, 52
Cocoa, 106, 138
Cocoa butter, 56, 138
Coconut water, 131, 133
Coconuts, 83, 134, 135
Coenzyme Q_{10} (CoQ_{10}), 59, 60,
    156–157
Coffee, 22
Colitis, ulcerative, 112, 113, 116–117,
    162, 163, 164
Collagen, 2, 9, 146, 159
Colon, 109, 110
Computed tomography (CT), 67
Constipation, 111, 160
Copper, 159
CoQ_{10}. *See* Coenzyme Q_{10} (CoQ_{10}).
Corticosteroids, 114
Crackers, raw, 123
Cramps, muscular, 79
C-reactive protein (CRP), 96
Crohn's disease, 65, 66, 78, 112, 113,
    163, 164
Crypts, 86
Cucumbers, 129, 130
Culturelle, 118
Curcumin, 84, 165–166
Cysteine, 51
Cystic duct, 57
Cystic fibrosis, 65

Dairy products, 142, 154, 157, 158
Dandelion root, 166
Darwin, Charles, 109
Defecation, 111
Dementia, 32
Dentures, 6, 15
Dermatitis, contact, 106
Dermatitis herpetiforms, 101
Desmosomes, 97

Detoxification, 47, 81–82
DGL (deglycyrrhized licorice). *See*
    Licorice.
Diabesity, 60
Diabetes, 14
    Type I, 76
    Type II, 49, 60, 76
Diaphragm, 23–24, 38
Diarrhea, 95, 111, 113
Diet, 52, 64, 80, 89, 121–126, 162
    elimination, 9, 124, 126
    excluded/included foods, 122–125
    gluten-free, 125
    isoflavone, 89
    high fat, low-carbohydrate (HFLC),
        52, 118, 121
    NeuroLipid Keto (ketogenic), 122
    paleo, 122
    specific carbohydrate (SCD), 122
    sulfur-containing, 89
    vegan, 89
    wheat-free, 125
Digestion, 4, 21, 27, 32, 77–78, 86,
    121
    nutritional plan, 121–142
    supplement plan, 143–164
Digestive algorithm, 120
Diseases, chronic, 1–2
Diverticula, 118, 119
Diverticular disease, 118–119
Diverticulitis, 118
Diverticulosis, 118
Dressings, salad, 124
Drinks, power/nutrient delivery,
    127–134
Dulse, 129
Duodenum, 37, 38, 49, 58, 70, 75, 85
Dysbiosis, 70, 71, 72, 85–92, 98–99,
    163
Dysphagia, 20

Easy Vegetable Power Drink, 130–131
Edema, 79
Egg protein powder, 128, 137, 138
Eggs, 123, 142, 159
Electrolytes, 100, 111, 127, 128, 131,
    148–149, 160

E-lyte Balanced Electrolyte Concentrate, 127, 128, 132, 136, 137, 148
Endoscopic retrograde cholangiopancreatography (ERCP), 67
Enzymes, 126, 148
    CYP450, 50
    Cytochrome P450 2E1 (CYP2E1), 81
    digestive, 69, 73, 76, 83, 86, 107, 149, 152
    pancreatic, 38, 76, 80, 84, 149, 151, 152–153
EPI. See Exocrine pancreatic insufficiency (EPI).
Esophagus, 18–19, 28, 60, 96, 161, 162
Estrogen, 63–64
Excitotoxins, 36
Excretion, 47–48, 49
Exercise, 36, 149
Exocrine pancreatic insufficiency (EPI), 77–78, 81, 83
Eyes, dry, 79

Fasts, 141
Fatigue, 79, 164
Fats, 21, 22, 38, 49, 58, 59, 70, 76, 121, 142, 165
    digestion of, 77, 79, 152
    saturated, 56, 134
    trans, 124
Fatty acid deficiency, 68–69
Fatty acids, 86, 115
Fatty liver, 48, 51, 52
Feces, 49, 110, 134
Feeding tubes, 34
Fermentation, 21, 22
Fiber, dietary, 33, 64, 119, 165
Fibric acid, 65
Fibrosis, 52, 81, 154
Fight or flight response, 26, 27
Fillings, dental, 13
Fish, 56, 63, 122–123
5Rs approach, 73, 125–126
Flatulence, 78
Flaxseed Tea, 141
Flour, 102, 105

Folate, 3, 8, 9, 32, 33, 88, 114, 116, 164
Folic acid. See Folate.
Food intolerances, 22, 29, 65, 82, 88, 104, 113, 154
Foods, 3, 8, 15, 22, 28, 121–125
    excluded/included in HFLC diet, 122–125
    fermented, 126, 133
    FODMAP, 126
    fried, 22
    genetically-modified, 101
    refined, 64, 124
    super, 134
Framington Heart Study, 32
Free radicals, 81, 145
Fructo and galacto-oligosaccharides, 126
Fructose, 126
Fruits, 124

Galland, Leo, 95, 97
Gallbladder, 28, 29, 37, 38, 49, 57–73, 76, 140–142
    relief recipes, 140–142
Gallstones, 49, 50, 53, 63–66, 80, 81, 142
    relief program, 165–166
GALT (Gut-associated lymphoid tissue), 94–95, 97
Garlic, 163
Gastic mucosa, 110
Gastric band surgery, 78
Gastrin, 38
Gastroesophageal reflux disease (GERD), 17–36, 37, 162
    causes, 21–22
    effects, 23
    supplements for, 156, 160–161
    symptoms, 19–20
Gastroesophageal sphincter. See Sphincters, cardiac.
Gastrointestinal (GI) tract, 4, 8
Gc-MAC, 35, 133–134
Gelatin, 131
GERD. See Gastroesophageal reflux disease (GERD).
Ginger, 135

Gingivitis, 13
Glucosamine, 105, 131
Glucose, 14, 64, 86, 135
Glucuronidation, 50
Glutamine, 101, 154–155
Glutathione, 51, 160
Gluten ataxia, 103
Gluten, 8, 9, 61–62, 99, 102–103, 113, 125, 142
Glycans, 95–96, 104, 105
Glycerides, 86
Glycerin, 137, 138
Glycine, 131
Go-to-Green Smoothie, 129–130
Grains, 124–125
Green Soup Recipe for Relief of Gallbladder Pain, 141
Gums, 5, 9, 12–15
    disease. See Periodontal disease.
Gut-associated lymphoid tissue. See GALT (Gut-associated lymphoid tissue).

H. pylori. See Helicobacter pylori.
Hashimoto's hypothyroidism, 73
Hazelnuts, 138
Heart disease, 8, 32, 44, 157
Heartburn, 19, 25
HeartMath, 161
Helicobacter pylori, 21, 37, 40–44, 78, 90, 162
    diagnosis, 42
    treatment, 42–43, 162
Hematochezia, 113
Hemophilia, 54
Hepatic duct, 57
Hepatic encephalopathy, 52
Hepatitis, 53–56
    acute, 53, 55
    chronic, 53, 54, 55–56
    fecal-oral transmission, 53, 54
    infectious, 51, 53–54
    intravenous drug needle transmission, 54
    sexual transmission, 54
    types, 53–55
Hepatocytes, 48

Hepotobiliary (HIDA) scan, 62
Herbs, bitter, 142
Hernias
    exercise and, 36
    hiatus, 23–32, 36
    mixed, 26
    rolling hiatus, 25–26
    sliding hiatus, 25, 29, 161
    strangulated, 26
Herpes gingivostomatits, 10
Herpes labialis, 10
Herpes simplex (HSV), 7, 10–11
HFLC. See Diet, high fat, low-carbohydrate (HFLC).
HHS/VNI. See Hiatus hernia syndrome/vagus nerve imbalance (HHS/VNI).
Hiatal hernia. See Hiatus hernia.
Hiatus, 24, 27
Hiatus hernia syndrome/vagus nerve imbalance (HHS/VNI), 26–28
    supplements for, 160–161
Hippocrates, 86
Homeostasis, 47, 48
Homocysteine, 31, 32, 33, 116
Hormones, 8, 13, 63–64, 69–70
HPV. See Human papilloma virus (HPV).
HSV. See Herpes simplex (HSV).
Human papilloma virus (HPV), 34
Hydrochloric acid. See Stomach acid.
Hydrogen breath test, 92
Hypochlorhydria, 21, 23, 31, 32–33, 72
Hypothyroidism, 71

IBD. See Inflammatory bowel disease (IBD).
Ileocecal valve, 109
Ileum, 85, 109
Immune system, 10, 13, 59, 60, 72, 86, 87, 94, 145, 148, 157, 159
Immune-gG, 126
Incisors, 6
Infections, 153, 158
Inflammation, 45, 52, 60, 61, 87, 96, 99, 105, 112, 114, 131, 145, 146, 162, 163, 166
    chronic, 13, 78

Inflammatory bowel disease (IBD), 13, 109, 111–118
   supplements for, 163–164
Influenza, 105
Insulin, 60, 64, 75
Insulin resistance, 52, 76
Interleukin 1, 7
Intestines, large, 109–120
   layers, 110
Intestines, small, 60, 78, 85–87, 93–97, 107, 112
   junctions, 87, 96–97, 98, 144
   supplements for, 149–155
   walls, 85–87, 99
Intrinsic factor, 32
Iodine, 2, 67, 73, 166
Iron, 3, 8, 9, 33, 55, 114, 116, 159
Irritable bowel syndrome (IBS), 119
Islets of Langerhans, 75

Jaundice, 50, 53, 58, 66
Jaws, 5
Jejunal feeding, 83
Jejunum, 85

Kale, 129, 130
Kane, Ed, 115
Kane, Patricia, 29, 115
Kefir, 123, 126, 128, 133
Kidneys, 105
Kissing, 7
Kiwi fruit, 130
Kozyrskyj, Anita, 71-72
Kuhne, Louis, 87

Lactase, 107
Lactobacillus bacteria, 87-88, 133
Lactose, 126
Lactose intolerance, 107
Lactose-mannitol challenge test, 88
Lampria propria, 110
Laparotomy, 68
Leaky gut, 47, 48, 87, 96–97, 97–101, 102, 144, 153, 154, 154
Lectins, 96, 104, 105
Legumes, 158
Lemon balm, 11

Lentils, 123
Leukoplakia, 12
Lichen planus, 12
Licorice, 9, 11, 156, 160
Linseeds. *See* Seeds, flax.
Linusit Gold, 127
Lipases, 76, 77
Lipids, 56, 60, 64, 105, 116
Liver, 37, 47–56, 57, 97, 165
   disorders, 49–56
   failure, 50–52
   stress, 98
Liver flukes, 66
Lobules, 48
Lower esophageal sphincter. *See* Sphincters, cardiac.
Lunch, 138–139
Lymphatic ducts, 94
Lysine, 11
Lysophosphatidylcholine (LPC), 117

Macrophage activating factor (MAF), 133–134
Magnesium, 79, 111, 131, 148, 160, 166
Magnetic resonance imaging (MRI), 67
Malabsorption, 72, 78, 89, 105, 115–116
Malnutrition, 3, 13, 52, 98, 113, 114, 115–116
MALT lymphoma (MALToma), 42
Marshall, Barry, 40
Mastic gum, 162
Mayonnaise, 124
Meals, 122, 138–139
Meal replacements, 127–128
Meat, 122, 157, 159
Medicine, 162
   Chinese, 6, 135
Medulla oblongata, 26
Melatonin, 84
Menstrual cycle, 64
Mercury, 28, 36, 73, 160
Mesentery, 112
Metabolic disorders, 59
Metabolic syndrome, 51, 52
Metabolism, first-pass, 47–48

Metals, heavy, 27, 31, 72, 73, 99, 160
Metchnikoff, Élie, 87
Methionine, 160
Methylation, 8, 33
Methylmalonic acid (MMA) test, 116
Methyltetrahydrolfolate (MTHF), 164
Micelles, 49, 77, 152
Microbiome, 89
Microflora, 88–92, 94
Microvilli, 86
Milk, 113, 123, 128, 142, 158
Mineralization, 2
Minerals, trace, 34
Mint, 139
Mitochondria, 60, 138, 156
Molars, 6
Monosaccharides, 87
Monosodium glutamate, 124, 125
Mouth, 1–15
    diseases, 7–15
    function, 4–7
    inside, 2–4, 5
    mucosal surface, 2–3, 5, 7
    palate, 5
Mucilage, 155
Mucin. See Mucus and mucous
    membranes.
Mucosal tolerance, 59
Mucous membranes. See Mucus and
    mucous membranes.
Mucus and mucous membranes,
    38–39, 44–45, 58, 59, 91, 95–96,
    97, 104–105, 111, 116, 119–120,
    122, 131, 153, 155, 156, 157,
    163
Mumps, 5
Murphy's sign, 72
Muscles, 79

NAC. See N-acetyl cysteine (NAC).
N-acetyl cysteine (NAC), 51, 56
N-acetyl glucosamine (NAG), 104, 105
NAFLD (Non-Alcoholic Fatty Liver
    Disease). See NASH (Non-
    Alcoholic Steato-Hepatitis).
NAG. See N-acetyl glucosamine (NAG).
NAPQI, 51

NASH (Non-Alcoholic Steato-
    Hepatitis), 48–49, 52, 82, 154
National Institutes of Health (NIH),
    41
Necrosis, 80
Nerves, 5, 10
    vagus, 5, 26, 32, 36, 38, 39, 110,
    142
Nervous system, 26, 27, 103
Neuralgia, 7
Neurolipid Cocktail, 35, 56, 119,
    127–128, 157, 164
Nickel, 73, 99, 106–107, 160
Nigella sativa, 43
Night blindness, 79
Nitrosamines, 82
NK kappa B (NFkB), 114–115
Non-Alcoholic Fatty Liver Disease.
    See NASH (Non-Alcoholic
    Steato-Hepatitis).
Non-Alcoholic Steato-Hepatitis. See
    NASH (Non-Alcoholic Steato-
    Hepatitis).
Nonsteroidal anti-inflammatory drugs
    (NSAIDs), 41, 44–45, 99, 116,
    153, 154
Noodles, 123
NSAIDs. See Nonsteroidal anti-
    inflammatory drugs (NSAIDs).
Nutrient deficiencies, 3–4, 6, 8, 13
Nuts, 119, 123, 135, 137, 138, 157,
    158

Obesity, 20, 22, 49, 52, 60, 64
Oils, 142, 157
    BodyBio Balance, 123, 128, 164
    coconut, 56, 130, 136
    essential, 134
    flaxseed, 140
    hemp, 123, 130
    olive, 56, 140
    oregano, 163
    peppermint, 11, 165
    sunflower, 130
Oleic acid, 56
Omega-3 fatty acids, 56, 115
Omega-6 fatty acids, 56, 115, 164

Omega-9 fatty acids, 56
Omeprazole, 43
Onions, 142
Oral health, 156–159
Orthophosphoric acid, 166
Osteopenia, 79, 116
Osteoporosis, 14, 116
Ox bile, 73
Oxidation, 50
Oxidative stress, 81, 145

Pancreas, 38, 75–84
   disorders, 77–84
Pancreatitis, 80–84
   acute, 80
   chronic, 80–84
   surgery for, 83
Paracetamol. See Acetaminophen.
Parasites, 90, 99, 153
   biliary, 62–63
Parasuicide, 50
Parsley, 138–139, 141
PC. See Phosphatidylcholine (PC).
Peanuts, 124
Pecans, 137
Pepsin, 19
Periodontal disease, 2, 3, 12–15
   supplements for, 156–160
Periodontal membrane, 2
Periodontitis, 13
Peripheral neuropathy, 79
Peristalsis, 19, 33–34, 60, 110, 111,
   134
Peritonitis, 40, 65, 119
Perm A vite, 126
Petrochemicals, 82
Peyer's patches, 94
pH, 32, 70, 90
Phosphate, 148
Phosphatidylcholine (PC), 56, 101,
   116–117, 160, 163–164, 165, 166
Phospholipids, 116–117, 121–122
Phosphorus, 114, 131
Piercings, 106
Plaque, dental, 13
Pollution, environmental, 81
Polymers, 96

Polyols, 126
Polysaccharides, 4, 87
Pork, 142
Porridge, 134–135
Potassium, 114, 148
Power bars, 137–138
Power Drink. See Neurolipid Cocktail.
PPIs. See Proton pump inhibitors
   (PPIs).
PQQ, 138
Prebiotics, 89
Pregnancy, 22
Premolars, 6
Preservatives, 8
Probiotics, 43, 73, 89, 101, 117–118,
   126, 133–134
Progesterone, 28, 64
Proline, 131
Prostheses, 106, 107
Proteases, 19, 76
Proteins, 3, 5, 21, 22, 32, 36, 76, 114,
   116, 157
Proton pump inhibitors (PPIs), 17–18,
   90
Psoriasis, 61, 73, 115
Pyloric sphincter. See Sphincters,
   pyloric.
Pyloroplasty, 27, 39
Pyridoxine. See Vitamin B_6.

Quercetin, 9
Quinoa, 138–139
Quinoa Tabbouleh, 138–139

Radiation, 34
Reams, Carey, 27
Rebound withdrawal, 4
Receptors, cell surface, 102
Recipes, 127–142
Rectum, 110, 111, 116–117
Reflux. See Gastroesophageal reflux
   disease (GERD).
Retina, 59
Rhodioloa, 161
Riboflavin. See Vitamin B_2.
Rochlitz, Steven, 26–28, 36
Roundworms, 62

Saccharomyces boulardii, 89
Salads, 123
Saliva, 4, 13, 14, 148
Salivary glands, 5
Schatzki ring, 28
Seats, 28
Secretin, 28, 38, 69, 70, 76
Secretory immunoglobulin A (SIgA),
      90–91
Seeds, 119, 123, 157, 158
   chia, 127, 134, 135, 155
   cream of, 127–128, 129
   flax, 127, 134, 135, 136, 137, 138,
      141, 155
   pumpkin, 127, 134, 135
   sesame, 127, 135, 137, 138
   sunflower, 127, 134, 135
Selenium, 160
Serous layer, 110
SIBO (small intestinal bacterial
      overgrowth), 23, 60, 73, 78, 88,
      89, 91–92, 98–99, 111
   supplements for, 163
Sinus, maxillary, 6
Sinusitis, 6
Sinusoids, 48
Skin, 59, 61, 73, 122, 155
Sleep, 84
Slippery elm, 155
Slow-Cooked Bone Broth, 131–132
Slow-Cooked Chicken Broth, 132
Small intestinal bacterial overgrowth.
      See SIBO (small intestinal
      bacterial overgrowth).
Smoking, 12, 22, 55, 81, 83, 84, 106,
      162
Smoothies, 129–130
Snacks, 122, 137–138
SNAS. *See* Systematic nickel allergy
      syndrome (SNAS).
Soaked Seed Cream, 127–128, 129
Sodium, 148
Soups, 131
   chicken, 132
   vegetable, 130, 141
Sphincters, 37
   anal, 110

cardiac, 18, 28
   pyloric, 27, 37, 85
Spinach, 129
Spine, 161
Sprue. *See* Celiac syndrome.
Stainless steel, 106
Staphylococcus aureus (MRSA), 42
Starches, 4, 76
Statins, 60
Steatorrhea, 79, 83, 86
Steinman, O. Arthur, 28
Stiff person syndrome, 103
Stomach, 37–39, 96
Stomach acid, 19, 21, 27, 32, 38, 39,
      41, 70, 76, 90, 135, 149, 150
   low. *See* Hypochlorhydria.
Stools. *See* Feces.
Strate, L. L., 119
Stress, 7, 10, 22, 29–32, 35, 90–91,
      161
Submucosa, 110
Sugars, 4–5, 64, 76, 124, 142, 162
Sulphation, 50
Super green powder, 129
Super Phosphozyme, 73, 166
Supplements, 126, 143–166
   for cancer, 161–162
   for digestive support, 149–153
   for gallstones, 165–166
   for gastric ulcers, 162
   for GERD, 160–161
   for inflammatory bowel disease,
      163–164
   for intestinal healing, 153–155
   for oral health, 156–160
   for SIBO, 163
Sweating, 149
Swedish bitters, 142
Sweetness, 4
Sylimarin, 165
Systematic nickel allergy syndrome
      (SNAS), 106

Tabbouleh, 138–139
Tagamet. *See* Cimetidne.
Tahini, 137, 138
Taste, loss of, 14, 148

Taurine, 59, 73, 166
Teas, 141
Teeth, 2, 5, 6–7, 156–160
    meridians, 6
Therapeutic nutritional intervention
    program, 125–126
Thermomix, 127
Thiamine. *See* Vitamin B$_1$.
33-mer, 102
Thrush, oral, 9–10
Thymus extracts, 11
Thymus gland, 11
Tingling, 164
Tobacco. *See* Smoking.
Tofu, 158
Tomatoes, 139
Tongue, 3, 5–6
Transit time, 60, 90, 92
Transketolase, 8
Trematodes, 62–63
Triglycerides, 51, 52, 64
    medium-chain, 83, 134
Trimethylglycine. *See* Betaine.
Turmeric, 84, 165–166

Ulcers, 39–40, 154, 156
    esophageal, 25
    gastric, 27, 162
    hemorrhage, 40
    peptic, 37
Ultrasound scans, 66–67

Vagotomy, 27, 39
Vegetables, 123, 124, 129–131, 132,
    138–141, 157, 158
    juicing, 131
Veins, 47, 48, 94
Villi, 78, 86, 94
Vinegar, apple cider, 35, 132
Vinyl chloride, 82
Viruses, 99, 145
Vitamin A, 12, 33, 33, 49, 59, 79,
    114, 157
Vitamin B-complex, 3, 79, 157, 161,
    166
Vitamin B$_1$, 8, 79
Vitamin B$_2$, 8

Vitamin B$_3$, 59
Vitamin B$_5$, 88
Vitamin B$_6$, 8, 11, 33, 166
Vitamin B$_{12}$, 3, 4, 8, 10, 32, 33, 56,
    88, 114, 116, 164
Vitamin C, 4, 5, 9, 11, 33, 34, 43, 56,
    59, 114, 136, 145–146, 159
Vitamin D, 14, 49, 59, 79, 100, 101,
    114, 116, 118, 126, 143–145,
    158
Vitamin E, 12, 33, 43, 49, 56, 59, 114,
    157, 165
Vitamin K, 49, 59, 79, 88, 114, 158
Vitamins
    fat-soluble, 49, 105, 114
    megadosing, 4
    multi- , 9
    overdosing, 4
Vitamix, 127, 135
VSL#3, 117

Wakefield, Andrew, 112
Walnuts, 134, 138
Warren, Robin, 40
WDEIA. *See* Wheat-dependent
    exercise-induced anaphylaxis
    (WDEIA).
Weight, 60, 64–65, 114, 116
WGA. *See* Wheat germ agglutinin
    (WGA).
Wheat, 82, 83, 99, 101–106, 125, 154
Wheat-associated diseases, 101–106
Wheat germ agglutinin (WGA),
    104–105, 125
Wheat-dependent exercise-induced
    anaphylaxis (WDEIA), 104

Xenoestrogens, 64

Yeasts, 90, 99
Yogurt, 123

Zinc, 8, 11, 14, 33, 52, 101, 107, 114,
    126, 147–148, 159, 160
    taste test, 147, 148
Zinc carnosine, 154, 160
Zucchini, 141

ABOUT THE AUTHORS

Damien Downing, M.D., is president of the British Society for Ecological Medicine and editor of the Journal of Nutritional and Environmental Medicine. He has undertaken pioneering work in the treatment of allergies, the link between behavioral disorders and nutrition, and light therapy and the treatment of chronic fatigue, autism, and attention deficit/hyperactivity disorder. Dr. Downing maintains a private practice in the UK focusing on nutritional and alternative therapies.

Anne Pemberton, PGCE, RGN started her career as a nurse, specializing in heart and lung surgery, and worked in intensive care unit with people needing temporary life support following major surgery. During this time she married and had two children, one of whom was diagnosed with autism, and began to have her own health issues. At thirty-six she returned to University majoring in psychology. Her PGCE in autism was supposed help her home school her autistic son. Instead, the course introduced her to a few key people who changed her career trajectory.

At the end of 1999 Anne was diagnosed with chronic fatigue syndrome and celiac disease. At this time she realized that her physical symptoms exactly the same as those her child experienced—the aches and pains of fibromyalgia, the incredible tiredness, foggy head, poor digestion, sensory hypersensitivity and psoriasis. Did they have the same condition? She found herself heavily involved in nutritional therapy, retrained at the Institute for Optimum Nutrition, and created a nutrition and lifestyle plan that gave both of them their lives back. Anne is the Director of a Master's degree course in nutritional therapy at The Northern College of Acupuncture in York, England, and is also an instructor on the course. Her passion is fueled by seeing her clients become empowered to control their own health and well-being, and seeing her students graduate and begin their own practice to further benefit society.